BestMasters

T0238490

Springer awards „BestMasters" to the best master's theses which have been completed at renowned universities in Germany, Austria, and Switzerland.

The studies received highest marks and were recommended for publication by supervisors. They address current issues from various fields of research in natural sciences, psychology, technology, and economics.

The series addresses practitioners as well as scientists and, in particular, offers guidance for early stage researchers.

Matthias Kaeding

Bayesian Analysis of Failure Time Data Using P-Splines

Springer Spektrum

Matthias Kaeding
Hamburg, Germany

BestMasters
ISBN 978-3-658-08392-2 ISBN 978-3-658-08393-9 (eBook)
DOI 10.1007/978-3-658-08393-9

Library of Congress Control Number: 2014958185

Springer Spektrum

Printed on acid-free paper

Springer Spektrum is a brand of Springer Fachmedien Wiesbaden
Springer Fachmedien Wiesbaden is part of Springer Science+Business Media
(www.springer.com)

Contents

List of Figures

List of Tables

1 Introduction

Failure time analysis is a form of regression analysis where the time until an event occurs is of interest. The event is generically referred to as failure in this thesis, the observational units are referred to as individuals.

Unlike most regression models the model is not formulated for the conditional expectation. Most regression models for failure time analysis are formulated in terms of the *hazard rate*, giving the risk of failure and will be defined precisely in the following. A general formulation for the hazard rate is (Cox and Oakes 1984, p. 70):

$$h(t|z_i,\boldsymbol{\beta}) = h_0(t)\rho(\beta_1 z_1 + ..., \beta_k z_k) = h_0(t)\rho(\eta_i).$$

Here, the *baseline hazard* $h_0(t)$ gives the hazard of an individual with standard conditions, corresponding to $\boldsymbol{z} = \mathbf{0}$, $\eta_i = \boldsymbol{z}_i^\top \boldsymbol{\beta}$ is the *linear predictor* and $\rho(\cdot)$ is a nonnegative function satisfying $\rho(0) = 1$. Splines allow the replacement of linear effects of the form $\boldsymbol{z}_i^\top \boldsymbol{\beta}$ in the linear predictor by more general functions. This is useful for flexible modeling of the baseline hazard, treating time formally like a covariate. A spline is a function consisting of local polynomials that are joined together at points in the domain of the covariate. Splines can be understood as a regression model: Every spline can be written as a weighted sum of *basis functions* depending on a covariate, hence a regression model where the regression coefficients are given by the weigths.

The aim of this thesis is to present Bayesian methods for models where either the hazard rate, covariates, or both are modeled via splines, in discrete and continuous time. B-spline basis functions in combination with a penalty to avoid overfitting (usually called P-splines) are the main building blocks used for modeling. P-splines have good numerical properties, and allow fast computation. Additionally, other useful basis functions for failure time analysis will be given. Failures are always assumed to be nonrecurrent. A fully Bayesian perspective using MCMC methods is taken.

1.1 Outline

This thesis is structured as follows. At first the basic concepts of failure time analysis are introduced. For the statistical analysis of failure time data, time is represented by a random variable which is characterized by quantities that are specific for failure time modeling. These quantities can be used to construct the likelihood by taking into account special properties of failure time data, such as *censoring*, which refers to failure times that are not fully observed. Next, two central model families are introduced; the relative risk and the log-location-scale model family. The subsequent chapter gives an overview of computational and inferential methods as they are relevant for model building. The chapter concludes with the introduction of Bayesian P-splines using the Gaussian likelihood as an example. The sampling scheme for Gaussian responses can be adjusted for the probit model for discrete time and the lognormal model for continuous time. Subsequently, models for the analysis of discrete time are introduced. Gibbs sampler for these models are categorized here by methods embedded in the generalized linear model (GLM) and the latent variable framework. Based on those frameworks efficient Bayesian sampling schemes can be constructed. From the GLM framework iteratively weighted least squares (IWLS) proposals based on fisher scoring for the Metropolis-Hastings algorithm can be derived. Many sampling schemes for models using P-splines were developed on the basis on IWLS proposals, including sampling schemes for continuous time models. Discrete time models are illustrated using data of unemployment durations. Subsequently, estimation for continuous time is described. The focus is on relative risk models but the lognormal and extensions based on will also be discussed. The methods are illustrated using a data set on crime-recidivism. As final chapter, a summary with outlook will be given.

1.2 Notation

In this thesis standard notation as often used in the literature is used. The distinction between a random variable Y and its realizations y will be made in the introductory chapters and ignored for the later chapters when the meaning is obvious. The conventions used in this thesis are listed here. Conditioning on parameters will often be surpressed for notational simplicity.

Symbol	Explanation
x	scalar
$\boldsymbol{x} = (x_1, ..., x_n)^\top$	vector
$\boldsymbol{X}$	matrix
$I[\cdot]$	indicator function
$\text{diag}(x_1, ..., x_n)$	diagonal matrix obtained from $\boldsymbol{x}$
$\text{bdiag}(\boldsymbol{A}, \boldsymbol{B})$	block diagonal matrix out of matrices $\boldsymbol{A}, \boldsymbol{B}$

The following table gives an overview over important fixed symbols.

Symbol	Explanation
$h(t)$	hazard rate
$H(t)$	cumulative hazard rate
$h_0(t)$	baseline hazard
$H_0(t)$	cumulative baseline hazard
$G(t)$	survivor function
$\mathscr{D}$	available data
$L(\boldsymbol{\theta}\|\mathscr{D})$	likelihood
v_i	censoring indicator
η	linear predictor

The following table gives an overview over the shorthand used for the distributions.

Distribution	Shorthand	Parameter
normal	$N(\mu, \sigma^2)$	expectation μ, variance σ^2
truncated normal	$TN_{(a,b)}(\mu, \sigma^2)$	expectation μ, variance σ^2, support (a,b)
lognormal	$LN(\mu, \sigma^2)$	location μ,shape σ
inverse gamma	$IG(\alpha, \beta)$	shape α, scale β
gamma	$G(\alpha, \beta)$	shape α, rate β
Poisson	$\mathscr{P}(\lambda)$	mean/variance λ
inverse Wishart	$IW(a, \boldsymbol{B})$	degrees of freedom a, scale matrix $\boldsymbol{B}$

2 Basic Concepts of Failure Time Analysis

2.1 Continuous Time

Time is represented by the nonnegative random variable T with cumulative density function

$$F(t) = P(T \leq t),$$

and density

$$f(t) = dF(t)/dt.$$

For failure time analysis, T is generally characterized by other quantities. The survivor function gives the probability that T exceeds t:

$$G(t) = P(T > t) = 1 - F(t).$$

It always holds that no individual has failed at $T = 0$

$$G(0) = 1, \tag{2.1}$$

and it is usually assumed that every subject will fail eventually

$$\lim_{t \to \infty} G(t) = 0. \tag{2.2}$$

Variables with survivor function not satisfying 2.2 are called defective, for those it follows that E[T]=∞. The probability of failure in the small interval [t,t+dt) can be approximated by $h(t)dt$ (Aalen et al. 2008, pp. 5–17). The function $h(t)$ is the hazard rate, defined as:

$$h(t) = \lim_{\Delta \to 0} \frac{P(t \leq T < t + \Delta | T \geq t)}{\Delta}. \tag{2.3}$$

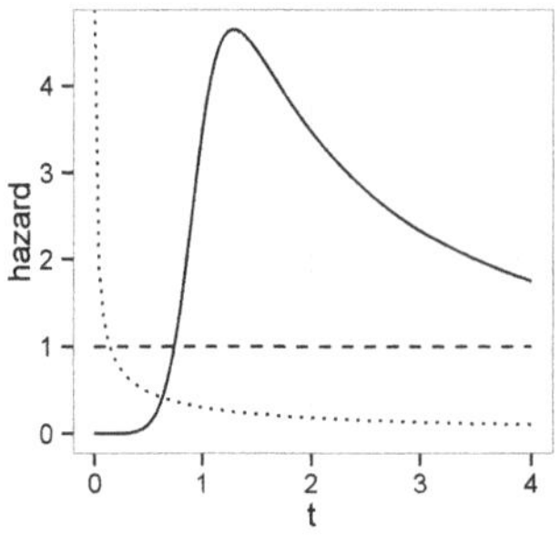

Figure 2.1: Some hazard rates

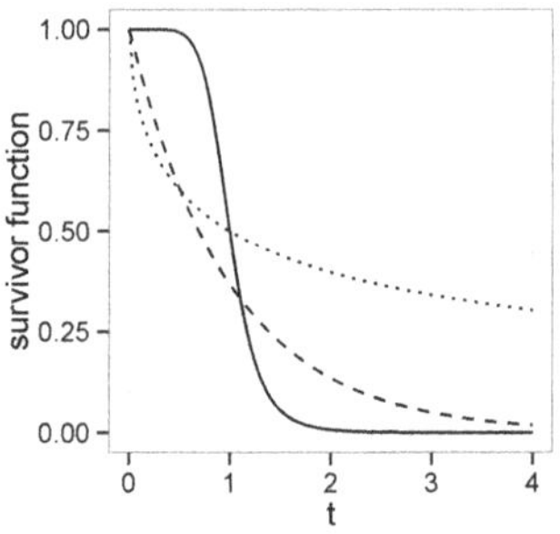

Figure 2.2: Some survivor functions

The probability $P(t \leq T < t+\Delta | T \geq t)$ is

$$\frac{F(t+\Delta) - F(t)}{G(t)}.$$

Hence 2.3 is

$$\frac{1}{G(t)} \lim_{\Delta \to 0} \frac{F(t+\Delta) - F(t)}{\Delta} = \frac{F'(t)}{G(t)} = \frac{f(t)}{G(t)},$$

showing that the hazard is a conditional density.

The cumulative hazard rate is

$$H(t) = \int_0^t h(t) = \int_0^t \frac{f(u)}{G(u)} du = [-\log G(u)]_0^t = -\log G(t),$$

due to 2.1. Hence, the survivor function can be written in terms of the hazard rate:

$$G(t) = \exp(-\int_0^t h(t)) = \exp(-H(t)). \tag{2.4}$$

The same applies for the density:

$$f(t) = h(t)G(t) = h(t)\exp(-H(t)).$$

Because of these relationships, the random variable T is fully specified by one of the given quantities. From 2.4, it can be seen that the function $h(t)$ only needs to satisfy

$$\int_0^t h(s)\,ds < \infty,$$

for all t and

$$\int_0^\infty h(s)\,ds = \infty$$

to be the hazard rate of a nondefective continuous variable (Kalbfleisch and Prentice 2002, p. 9). Many models in failure time modeling are formulated in terms of the hazard rate first.

2.2 Discrete Time

In the case of grouped failure times, an unobservable continous random variable $T^\star$ is partitioned into m+1 intervals $[a_0 = 0, a_1), [a_1, a_2), ..., [a_m, a_{m+1} = \infty)$, (Lawless 2003, p. 370). Observed are discrete failure times from the random variable $T = \{1, 2, .., m+1\}$, so that T$=t$ corresponds to T$^\star \in [a_{t-1}, a_t)$. The hazard in terms of T is

$$h(t) = P(T = t | T \geq t) = \frac{P(T = t)}{P(T \geq t)} = \frac{f(t)}{G(t-1)}. \tag{2.5}$$

Expressing 2.5 in terms of $T^\star$ gives:

$$h(t) = \frac{G^\star(a_t) - G^\star(a_{t-1})}{G^\star(a_t)} = 1 - \exp(-\int_{a_{t-1}}^{a_t} h^\star(u)\,du).$$

This is the probability of failure in interval t, conditional on reaching the interval. A discrete time model can be specified in terms of T or T*. Failure after interval t is a result of a sequence of binary trials unfolding in time (Kalbfleisch and Prentice 2002, p. 9):

$$G(t) = P(T > t) = P(T \neq 1 \cap T \neq 2 ... \cap T \neq t) =$$

$$P(T \neq 1)P(T \neq 2|T \neq 1)P(T \neq 3|T \neq 1, T \neq 2)...P(T \neq t|T \neq 1, ..., T \neq t-1).$$

The probability $P(T \neq x | T \neq x-1)$ is given by $1 - h(x)$, it follows that in analogy to the continuous case the survivor function can be expressed in terms of the hazard rate:

$$G(t) = \prod_{j=1}^{t} (1 - h(j)).$$

Assuming grouped failure times might not be appropriate in all cases, as some random variables are intrinsically discrete. Some helpful results follow from this assumption however, and estimation is easier by deriving inferences on the likelihood contributions following from 2.2, leading to an identical modeling framework.

2.3 Likelihood Construction

Failure time data have some special characteristics which have to be accounted for in the construction of the likelihood. A failure time is referred to as censored when the actual failure time is not observed but it is only known to fall into an interval. Failure times are *left-truncated* if they are only observable if they exceed a truncation time. Time varying covariates are often available in the data set. In the following sections, based on Klein and Moeschberger (2003, pp. 63-77), it will be clarified how these conditions are accounted for in the formulation of the likelihood. Conceptually, these adjustments can be represented in an unified framework by varying the likelihood contributions. As a consequence, the likelihood becomes more difficult to work with but there are computational methods which simplify estimation.

2.3.1 Censoring and Truncation

In the presence of right-censoring, the observed failure time for an individual is

$$t_i = \min(\dot{t}_i, c_i).$$

Here, $\dot{t}_i$ is the true failure time and c_i is the censoring time. The indicator variable v_i is defined as

$$v_i = \begin{cases} 1 & \text{if } \dot{t}_i \leq c_i, \\ 0 & \text{if } \dot{t}_i > c_i, \end{cases}$$

and is usually referred to as censoring indicator. The available data is given by:

$$D = \{(t_i, \delta_i, \mathbf{z}_i^\top)_{i=1}^n\}.$$

Here, $\mathbf{z}_i = (z_{i1}, z_{i2}, ..)^\top$ is the vector of covariates of individual i. To proceed, it is necessary to make assumptions about the process generating the censoring times. Under the assumption of *random censoring*, $C_1, ..., C_n$ are i.i.d. random variables with survivor function S() and pdf s() depending on $\boldsymbol{\phi}$, independent of $T_1, ..., T_n$ and each other. Let $\boldsymbol{\theta}$ be the parameter vector of interest on which the survivor function of $T_1, ..., T_n$ depends. Under random censoring, the full likelihood contribution $L_i^\star$ is

$$L_i^\star = G(t_i|\mathbf{z}_i) = P(T_i > t_i|\mathbf{z}_i)s(t_i)$$

for a right-censored failure time and

$$L_i^\star = G(t_i|\mathbf{z}_i)h(t_i|\mathbf{z}_i)S(t_i) = f(t_i|\mathbf{z}_i)S(t_i)$$

for a completely observed failure time. Under *noninformative censoring*, we have $G(t_i|\boldsymbol{\theta}, \boldsymbol{\phi}) = G(t_i|\boldsymbol{\theta})$. Further we assume that $T_1, ..., T_n$ are i.i.d. or independent given the covariates. Under those assumptions, the likelihood is given by:

$$\begin{aligned} L(\boldsymbol{\theta}|D) &= c\prod_{i=1}^n h(t_i|\mathbf{z}_i, \boldsymbol{\theta})^{v_i} G(t_i|\mathbf{z}_i, \boldsymbol{\theta}) \\ &\propto \prod_{i=1}^n L_i, \end{aligned}$$

where $c = \prod_{i=1}^n S(t_i)^{v_i} s(t_i)^{1-v_i}$ is a multiplicative constant and

$$L_i = h(t_i|\mathbf{z}_i, \boldsymbol{\theta})^{v_i} G(t_i|\mathbf{z}_i, \boldsymbol{\theta}).$$

For Bayesian analysis, the assumption $f(\boldsymbol{\theta}, \boldsymbol{\phi}) = f(\boldsymbol{\theta})f(\boldsymbol{\phi})$ is also necessary so that $f(\boldsymbol{\phi})$ factors out of the posterior. In this thesis it is always assumed that censoring is random and noninformative. For discrete failure time data a failure indicator y is introduced for every interval before and including the failure time, so that $P(y_{ij} = h(j|z_i))$:

$$y_{ij} = \begin{cases} 1 & \text{if individual i fails in interval } [a_{j-1}, a_j), \\ 0 & \text{if } t_i > a_j. \end{cases}$$

Assuming that censoring occurs at the end of the interval, the likelihood contribution of an uncensored and a right-censored individual respectively equal

$$\prod_{i=1}^{t_i} P(y_{ij} = 0)^{1-y_{ij}} P(y_{ij} = 1)^{y_{ij}} = h(t_i|z_i) \prod_{i=1}^{t_{i-1}} (1 - h(i|z_i)) =$$
$$h(t_i|z_i) G(t_i - 1|z_i) = f(t_i|z_i),$$

and

$$\prod_{i=1}^{t_i} P(y_{ij} = 0) = \prod_{i=1}^{t_i} (1 - h(j|z_i)) = G(t_i|z_i).$$

The likelihood is:

$$L(\theta|D) = \prod_{i=1}^{n} \prod_{j=1}^{t_i} (1 - h(j|z_i))^{1-y_{ij}} h(j|z_i)^{y_{ij}},$$

which is the likelihood of a Bernoulli distribution. The same result would have been obtained for an intrinsically discrete random variable. Discrete failure times can be analyzed by methods for this distribution. In practice, this is achieved by changing a data set given in the usual form for failure time analysis 2.1 into the longitudinal form 2.2. Under interval censoring, it is only known that failure occurred during the interval $[l_i, r_i)$. Interval-censoring can be viewed as generalization of right-censoring, the interval corresponding to right-censoring is $[l_i, \infty)$, while by

Table 2.1: Discrete data

id	t	z1	v
1	3	9	1
2	2	12	0

Table 2.2: Discrete data - longitudinal

id	y	z1
1	0	9
1	0	9
1	1	9
2	0	12
2	0	12

convention the interval of a uncensored individual is $[l_i = t_i, r_i = t_i)$. For continuous time, the interval can be set to $(l_i, r_i]$ $[l_i, r_i]$ or (l_i, r_i) as the same information about the failure time is represented (Sun 2006, p. 15), this is not true for discrete time. In this thesis, the notation $[l_i, r_i)$ is used. Grouped failure times are a special case of interval-censoring where all no intervals overlap (Lawless 2003, p. 64). The available data is given by

$$D = \{([l_i, r_i), \mathbf{z}_i^\top)_{i=1}^n\}.$$

The likelihood contribution is given by:

$$L_i = P(l_i \leq T_i < r_i | \mathbf{z}_i) = G(l_i | \mathbf{z}_i) - G(r_i | \mathbf{z}_i).$$

Under left-truncation, a failure time can only be observed if it exceeds a truncation time tr_i. Analysis of those cases proceeds by conditioning on failure after tr_i. For example, for continuous time, the contribution of an uncensored, left-truncated individual is:

$$\begin{aligned}\frac{f(t_i|\mathbf{z}_i)}{S(tr_i|\mathbf{z}_i)} &= \frac{h(t|\mathbf{z}_i)\exp(-\int_0^{t_i} h(t|\mathbf{z}_i)\,dt}{\exp(-\int_0^{tr_i} h(t|\mathbf{z}_i)\,dt} \\ &= h(t|\mathbf{z}_i)\exp(-\int_{tr_i}^{t_i} h(t|\mathbf{z}_i)\,dt.\end{aligned}$$

For discrete time:

$$\frac{f(t_i|z_i)}{S(tr_i|z_i)} = \frac{h(t_i|z_i)\prod_{j=1}^{t_i-1}(1-h(j|z_i))}{\prod_{j=1}^{tr_i}(1-h(j|z_i))} = h(t_i|z_i)\prod_{j=tr_i+1}^{t_i-1}(1-h(j|z_i)),$$

so conveniently by deleting failure indicators up to and including the truncation time, the likelihood contribution is correct. Combining the concepts, the data is given by

$$\{(l_i, r_i, tr_i, z_i)_{i=1}^n\}.$$

2.3.2 Time Varying Covariates

For covariates depending on time a distinction must be made between *internal* and *external* covariates (Kalbfleisch and Prentice 2002, pp. 196–199): For the former case it holds that

$$h(t|\mathbf{Z}(t), \boldsymbol{\beta}, T \geq u) = h(t|\mathbf{Z}(t), \boldsymbol{\beta}, T = u), 0 < u \leq t,$$

this implies that the covariates $\mathbf{Z}(t)$ affect the hazard, but failure does not affect the covariate path $\mathbf{Z}(t)$. Internal covariates are those that are directly involved with failure: As such, $G(t|\mathbf{Z}(t), \boldsymbol{\beta})$ can no longer be interpreted as a survivor function. Inclusion of internal covariates is problematic and here attention is restricted to external covariates. For example in the context of unemployment durations, an example of an internal covariate would be the amount of unemployment benefits an individual receives. Given that the amount is > 0 at month t, we have[1] $G(T > t|\mathbf{Z}(t)) = 1$. A (strictly seen, approximate) external variable might be the current rate of unemployment. Treatment of time varying covariates proceeds by taking them to be a stochastic process, an important property of which is *predictability*; informally, covariates are predictable if the values which explain variation in the hazard rate at time t are (to the researcher) known at an infinitesimal short moment before t (Berg 2001). The author gives as an example the case of an individual making a decision, e.g. accepting a job offer, under the anticipation of

[1] A model could in fact not even be fit with usual procedures here because of perfect seperation.

the realization of T. If this is unknown to the analyst, predictability is not given. In this thesis it is always assumed that covariates are predictable. Under this assumption - given regularity conditions - standard methods can be used with time varying covariates for relative risk models introduced in the next section.

While general sampling paths are possible for $\mathbf{Z}(t)$, changes in covariates values are usually observed at discrete points $(t_0 = 0 < t_1 < ... < t_{n_{i,k}})$. The survivor function of an individual can be written as product of conditional survivor functions without changing the likelihood:

$$
\begin{aligned}
G(t_i|z_i(t)) = \exp\{-\int_0^t h(u|z_i(u))\,du\} = \exp\{-\int_{t_0}^{t_1} h(u|z_i(u))\,du - \\
\int_{t_1}^{t_2} h(u|z_i(u))\,du - \ldots - \int_{t_{n_k}-1}^{t_{n_{i,k}}} h(u|z_i(u))\,du\} \\
= \prod_{j=1}^{n_{i,k}} G(t_j|t_j > t_{j-1}, z_i(j)).
\end{aligned}
$$

Every term $G(t_j|t_j > t_{j-1}, z_i(j))$ is the likelihood contribution of an right-censored individual with covariate $z_i(j)$ and failure time t_j left-truncated at t_{j-1}. As a consequence, the data set can be adjusted by a process called *episode splitting* (Blossfeld and Rohwer 2002, pp. 140–142), which can be seen in table 2.3. On the left is the

Table 2.3: Episode splitting

id	t	v	z1	tl	id	t	v	z1	z2	tl
1	5	1	3	0	1	3	0	3	11	0
2	7	0	5	0	1	5	1	3	15	3
					2	2	0	5	9	0
					2	5	0	5	4	2
					2	7	0	5	6	5

data set before, on the right the data set after episode splitting. After the split, the time varying covariate z_2 can be included. For discrete time, time-varying covariates can be inluded by varying the covariate values across the intervals.

2.4 Relative Risk and Log-Location-Scale Family

The Cox model or relative risk model, due to Cox (1972) is probably the most often used model for failure time modeling in continuous time. For models belonging to the relative risk family, the hazard rate is specified as:

$$h(t|\boldsymbol{z}(t),\boldsymbol{\beta}) = h_0(t)\exp(\boldsymbol{\beta}^T\boldsymbol{z}(t)), \tag{2.6}$$

implying a loglinear model for the hazard rate:

$$\log h(t|\boldsymbol{z}(t),\boldsymbol{\beta}) = \log h_0(t) + \boldsymbol{z}(t)^\top\boldsymbol{\beta}.$$

Here, the hazard rate consists of the baseline hazard $h_0(t)$, corresponding to $\boldsymbol{z} = \boldsymbol{0}$ on which the covariates act multiplicatively by $\exp(\boldsymbol{\beta}^\top\boldsymbol{z}(t))$. For time-constant covariates the model 2.6 is also known as proportional hazards model. In this case, the ratio of hazards of two individuals with covariate vectors $\boldsymbol{z}_i$ and $\boldsymbol{z}_j$ is

$$\frac{h_i(t|\boldsymbol{z}_i,\beta)}{h_j(t|\boldsymbol{z}_j,\beta)} = \frac{h_0(t)\exp(\boldsymbol{\beta}^\top\boldsymbol{z}_i)}{h_0(t)\exp(\boldsymbol{\beta}^\top\boldsymbol{z}_j)} = \exp(\boldsymbol{\beta}^\top(\boldsymbol{z}_i - \boldsymbol{z}_j)), \tag{2.7}$$

so $h_i(t|\boldsymbol{z}_i) \propto h_j(t|\boldsymbol{z}_j)$, independent of t. A one unit change in covariate z_p - given the other covariates are fixed - corresponds to multiplication of the hazard rate by the factor $\exp(\beta_p)$. This factor is also called the *hazard ratio* or *relative risk* of covariate p (Aalen et al. 2008, p. 9) as it gives the ratio 2.7 if $\boldsymbol{z}_i - \boldsymbol{z}_j = (0,..,0,1,0,..,0)^\top$, where the one is in position p. Frequentist inference is often based on the partial likelihood, which is free of the baseline hazard:

$$L_p(\beta|\mathscr{D}) = \prod_{i=1}^{d} \frac{\exp(z_i\boldsymbol{\beta})}{\sum_{j\in\mathscr{R}(i)}\exp(z_j\boldsymbol{\beta})}, \tag{2.8}$$

$t_{(1)}, t_{(2)}, ..., t_{(d)}$ are the ordered failure times and

$$\mathscr{R}(x) = \{i : t_i \geq x\}$$

is the risk set at time x. The estimator derived by maximization of 2.8 has properties that are very close to the optimality of maximum likelihood estimators. This - in addition to the simplicity of the model - explains the central role hold by the relative risk model in failure time modeling. As shown by Kalbfleisch (1979) by marginalizing over the baseline hazard a marginal posterior proportional to the partial likelihood is obtained if a gamma process - a stochastic process with gamma distributed increments - is used as prior for H_0 . Much literature on Bayesian failure time analysis is based on this approach - under which the baseline hazard is mainly viewed as nuisance parameter to be averaged over - motivated by the properties of the partial likelihood. This thesis is instead concerned with models based on the full posterior where the baseline hazard is estimated from the data. In this thesis, extensions of the basic Cox model with the following properties are discussed:

- The baseline hazard is either completely specified or the log-baseline is flexibly modeled via P-splines so that inferences are always based on the full posterior.
- Effects of the form $z_{ij}^{\top}\beta_j$ can be generalized to smooth functions $f_j(z_{ij})$.
- Time-dependent covariates and time-dependent effects can be included so that the often restrictive proportionality property is not satisfied.

Including these extensions is much easier working with the full posterior instead of the partial posterior (Fahrmeir et al. 2013, p. 430). Furthermore, very often an estimate of the baseline hazard is needed - e.g. for the prediction of survival probabilites - or the shape of the baseline hazard is of main interest. For example in econometric applications, there is often great interest if negative $(dh(t)/dt < 0)$ or positive $(dh(t)/dt > 0)$ duration dependence prevails (Heckman and Singer 1984).

Another important model family for continuous time is the log-location-scale family (Lawless 2003, pp. 26–28). It consists of distributions where $Y = \log T$ can be written as

$$Y = \log T = \mu + \sigma W,$$

where μ is a location parameter, for regression analysis taken as $\mathbf{Z}^\top\boldsymbol{\beta}$, σ is a scale parameter and W has density f_0, belonging to the location-scale family of the form

$$f_W(y) = \frac{1}{\sigma} f_0(\frac{y-\mu}{\sigma}).$$

By the relation 2.4 regression coefficients can be interpreted directly as marginal effects in terms of the conditional expectation of Y, or in terms of T via the factor $\exp(\beta_j)$. The effect of z_j is to accelerate or slow down time until failure, therefore models of this form are also called accelerated failure time models (AFT). This effect can be understood to be relative to an individual with covariate vector $\mathbf{0}$. The survivor function of T can be represented in terms of the survivor Function of W, denoted G_0 in analogy to the relative risk model, as it corresponds to $\mathbf{z}_i = \mathbf{0}$:

$$P(T > t|z, \boldsymbol{\beta}) = P(\exp(\mathbf{Z}^\top\boldsymbol{\beta})\exp(\sigma W)) > t)$$
$$= P(W > \frac{\log t - \mu}{\sigma}) = G_0(\frac{\log t - \mu}{\sigma}).$$

The only intersection of the log-location and relative risk family is the Weibull distribution and by proxy the exponential distribution, which is a special case of the Weibull.

This thesis is focused mainly on the relative risk family and only inference for the lognormal (and some extensions based on it) and the Weibull distribution from the family is discussed. For the lognormal model discussion is restricted to time-constant covariates and time-constant effects as inclusion of those is a very specialized topic and rarely done, but inclusion of smooth effects $f_j(z_{ij})$ will be discussed.

3 Computation and Inference

Bayesian inference is based on the posterior distribution of the parameters $\boldsymbol{\theta} = (\theta_1, \theta_2, ...)^\top$, given by

$$f(\boldsymbol{\theta}|\mathscr{D}) = cL(\boldsymbol{\theta}|\mathscr{D})f(\boldsymbol{\theta}),$$

with normalizing constant $c = [\int L(\boldsymbol{\theta}|\mathscr{D})f(\boldsymbol{\theta})\,d\boldsymbol{\theta}]^{-1}$. In rare cases c can be given in closed form. In most cases the posterior distribution can not be normalized and inference is based on a simulation of the posterior distribution, usually obtained via Markov chain simulation Monte Carlo (MCMC) methods.

The purpose of this chapter is to give an overview over computational and inferential methods relevant for this thesis.

3.1 MCMC

Following Roberts (1996, pp. 205–209) a Markov chain is a sequence of random variables $X_0, X_1, ...$ where the distribution of X_t given $X_{t-1}, X_{t-2}, ..., X_0$ only depends on X_{t-1}, so that

$$X_t|X_{t-1}, X_{t-2}, ..., X_0 \sim K(X_t|X_{t-1}).$$

The conditional probability density $K(X_t|X_{t-1})$ is referred to as transition kernel. If the marginal distribution of X_{t+1} is π, so that

$$\int K(X_{t+1}|X_t)\pi(X_t)\,dX_t = \pi(X_{t+1})$$

holds (given that $X_t \sim \pi$), the chain has *stationary* distribution π; implying that if one sample is obtained from π, all subsequent samples are from π. For this to be the case the transition kernel has to allow free moves over the state space. For Bayesian inference the transition kernel is chosen so that π equals the posterior

Algorithm 1: Metropolis-Hastings algorithm

1. Choose start values $(\boldsymbol{\theta}_1^{(0)}, ..., \boldsymbol{\theta}_k^{(0)})$
2. Draw a proposal $\boldsymbol{\theta}^\star$ from $g(\boldsymbol{\theta}^\star|\boldsymbol{\theta}^{(s-1)})$
3. Set $\boldsymbol{\theta}^{(s+1)} = \boldsymbol{\theta}^\star$ with probability $\alpha(\boldsymbol{\theta}^{(s-1)}, \boldsymbol{\theta}^\star), \boldsymbol{\theta}^{(s-1)})$ and $\boldsymbol{\theta}^{(s+1)} = \boldsymbol{\theta}^{(s)}$ with probability 1-$\alpha(\boldsymbol{\theta}^{(s-1)}, \boldsymbol{\theta}^\star)$, where
$$\alpha(\boldsymbol{\theta}^{(s-1)}, \boldsymbol{\theta}^\star) = \min\left(1, \frac{\pi(\boldsymbol{\theta}^\star|y)g(\boldsymbol{\theta}^{(s-1)}|\boldsymbol{\theta}^\star)}{\pi(\boldsymbol{\theta}^{(s-1)}|y)g(\boldsymbol{\theta}^\star|\boldsymbol{\theta}^{(s-1)})}\right)$$
4. Set s=s+1 and move to step 2

distribution.

If certain properties are met by the chain, averages $S^{-1}\sum_{i=1}^{S} h(x_i)$, where S denotes the chainlength, converge to expectation $E_\pi[h(X_i)]$. These properties - which for the methods used here are usually met - and deeper coverage of MCMC theory are given e.g. in Tierney (1996) or Robert and Casella (2004).

3.1.1 Metropolis-Hastings

The Metropolis-Hastings (MH) algorithm is an algorithm that allows samling from a density that is only known up to a proportionality constant. In pseudocode type notation, the algorithm is given by algorithm 1. Proportionality constants that are independent of $\boldsymbol{\theta}$ cancel out in the ratio $\alpha(\cdot,\cdot)$ and need not to be known. The transition kernel of the MH-algorithm at iteration s decomposes into a term corresponding to acceptance, and a term corresponding to rejection of a draw:

$$\begin{aligned} K(X^{(t+1)}|X^{(t)}) =& \pi(X^{(t+1)}|X^\star)\alpha(X^{(t+1)}, X^\star) + \\ & I[X^{(s+1)} = X^\star]\{1 - \int \alpha(X^{(t+1)}, X^\star)\pi(X^\star|X^{(t)})\,dX^\star\}. \end{aligned}$$

It can be shown that

$$\pi(X^t)K(X^\star|X^{(t)}) = \pi(X^\star)K(X^{(t)}|X^\star) \tag{3.1}$$

Algorithm 2: Gibbs sampler

1 Choose start values $(\boldsymbol{\theta}_1^{(0)}, ..., \boldsymbol{\theta}_k^{(0)})$

2

$$\begin{aligned}
\text{sample } \boldsymbol{\theta}_1^{(s)} &\sim f(\boldsymbol{\theta}_1 | \boldsymbol{\theta}_2^{(s-1)}, ..., \boldsymbol{\theta}_k^{(s-1)}, \mathscr{D}) \\
\text{sample } \boldsymbol{\theta}_2^{(s)} &\sim f(\boldsymbol{\theta}_2 | \boldsymbol{\theta}_1^{(s)}, \boldsymbol{\theta}_3^{(s-1)}, ..., \boldsymbol{\theta}_k^{(s-1)}, \mathscr{D}) \\
&\vdots \\
\text{sample } \boldsymbol{\theta}_k^{(s)} &\sim f(\boldsymbol{\theta}_k | \boldsymbol{\theta}_1^{(s)}, ..., \boldsymbol{\theta}_{k-1}^{(s)}, \mathscr{D})
\end{aligned}$$

3 Set s=s+1 and move to step 2

holds. By integrating 3.1 in X_t it can be proofed that the stationary distribution is π:

$$\int \pi(X^t) K(X^\star | X^{(t)}) = \pi(X^\star).$$

The choice of proposal density is crucial for the speed of convergence and the *mixing* of the chain (Rosenthal 2011): A Markov chain with transition kernel P_1 mixes faster compared to a Markov chain with transition kernel P_2 if $E_{P_1}(X_n - X_{n-1})^2 > E_{P_2}(X_n - X_{n-1})^2$. Faster mixing also implies lower variance for functionals of π as autocorrelation is lower. In general there is a tradeoff between high acceptance rates and good coverage of the parameter space (Gamerman and Lopes 2006, p. 196). A method to bypass this tradeoff is to use a proposal density that approximates the target distribution. Here, a high acceptance rate is an indicator for a good approximation. Most Metropolis-Hastings sampler used in this thesis take this approach.

3.1.2 Gibbs Sampler

To obtain a sample of $\boldsymbol{\theta}$ from π, the Gibbs sampler proceeds by sequentially sampling from the full conditional distributions of parameter blocks $\boldsymbol{\theta}_i, i = 1, ..., k$ formed from $\boldsymbol{\theta}$. The Gibbs sampler is given by algorithm 2. For the full conditional distribution of block i conditional on $\boldsymbol{\theta}$ excluding $\boldsymbol{\theta}_i$ the notation $f(\boldsymbol{\theta}_i | \cdot, \mathscr{D})$

will be used. The Gibbs sampler can be seen as a special case of the MH-algorithm, in which the proposal distribution for $\boldsymbol{\theta}_i$ is the full conditional distribution. Inserting $f(\boldsymbol{\theta}_i|\cdot,\mathscr{D})$ in $\alpha(\boldsymbol{\theta}^{(\star)}|\boldsymbol{\theta}^{(s-1)})$ gives an acceptance probability of 1 for all i. Optimally the blocks consist of correlated parameters.

For some (conditional conjugate) distributions draws from $f(\boldsymbol{\theta}_i|\cdot,\mathscr{D})$ can be obtained directly. For conditional distribution for which this is not the case a Metropolis-Hastings subchain can be used to obtain draws from the full conditionals. This will be often the case for the models in this thesis. A subchain of length one is sufficient, as for this choice the joint distribution converges to the stationary distribution, and further exploration of the full conditional would not necessarily accelerate convergence (Robert and Casella 2004, p. 393).
An important type of Gibbs sampler for failure time modeling is based on the data augmentation algorithm by Tanner and Wong (1987). Here, the parameter space is augmented by latent variables $Z_1,...,Z_p$ so that

$$f(\boldsymbol{\theta}|\mathscr{D}) = \int g(\boldsymbol{\theta},\mathbf{Z}|\mathscr{D})d\mathbf{Z},$$

holds, so $f(\boldsymbol{\theta}|\mathscr{D})$ can be expressed as $E_{\mathbf{Z}}[g(\boldsymbol{\theta},\mathbf{Z}|\mathscr{D})]$. The pdf $g(\boldsymbol{\theta},\mathbf{Z}|\mathscr{D})$ is called a completion of $f(\boldsymbol{\theta}|\mathscr{D})$. There are infinite possible completitions for a given density, g is chosen so that sampling from the full conditionals $g(\boldsymbol{\theta}_i|\mathbf{Z},\mathscr{D})$ is simplified (Robert and Casella 2004, p. 374). Completion Gibbs sampler are often used for missing data problems where $g(\cdot|\mathscr{D})$ is taken as $f(y_{observed}, y_{missing}|\mathscr{D})$. Censoring can be seen as special case of missing data, where the available data provides information about the range of missing values (Sun 2006, p. 249). Another important application for data augmentation are discrete failure time models, where the latent data is given by an underlying continuous variable, determining the value of the binary indicator.

3.2 Inference from Simulation Output

The simulation of the posterior distribution must be summarized in an appropriate manner. Point estimators for a parameter $\theta \in \Theta$ can be motivated from decision theory by defining a loss function $L(\gamma, \theta)$, and minimizing the posterior expected loss

$$\int_{\Theta} L(\gamma, \theta) f(\theta|\mathscr{D}) d\theta. \tag{3.2}$$

It can be shown that the minimizer of 3.2 equals the minimizer of the integrated risk

$$\int_{\Theta} \int_{\mathscr{X}} f(x|\theta) L(q(x), \theta) dx f(\theta) d\theta,$$

where $x \in \mathscr{X}$ and $q(x)$ is an estimate of θ.

Table 3.1: Loss functions and corresponding estimators

$L(\gamma, \theta)$	Bayes estimator
$(\theta - \gamma)^2$	Posterior mean
$\|\theta - \gamma\|$	Posterior median
$I[\gamma \neq \theta]$	Posterior mode[1]

Such a minimizer is called a *Bayes estimator* (Robert 2001, pp. 52–54). Different loss functions correspond to different Bayes estimators. The most common ones are given in table 3.1. The corresponding Bayes estimators can be obtained from MCMC output as empirical counterpart.

To communicate estimation uncertainty the interval containing $100(1-\alpha)\%$ of the posterior density is often reported. This interval can be directly obtained from MCMC output, invariant to one-to-one transformations of the parameter, and is directly interpretable. An alternative is the set of highest posterior density, for a given α defined as the set $C = \{\theta \in \Theta : f(\theta|\mathscr{D}) \geq k(\alpha)\}$, where $k(\alpha)$ is the largest constant satisfying

$$f(C|\mathscr{D}) \geq 1 - \alpha$$

(Carlin and Louis 2011, p. 49). C is more difficult to determine but usually gives a shorter interval (given that the set can be described as interval). MCMC output is correlated, a measure for the resulting loss in precision is given by the effective sample size n_{eff} (Kass et al. 1998). This measure would equal the number of draws

[1]More precise, the corresponding loss function is defined as a sequence of losses, as $\int_{\Theta} I[\gamma \neq \theta] \pi(\theta|x) = 1$ (Robert 2001, p. 166).

if there would be no autocorrelation. It is defined as:

$$n_{eff} = \frac{S}{1+2\sum_{t=1}^{\infty}\rho_t}, \tag{3.3}$$

where ρ_t is the autocorrelation at lag t. A simple method to estimate the denominator of 3.3 is to use all empirical autocorrelations larger than a cutoff, say 0.1 (Carlin and Louis 2011, p. 151). Furthermore convergence of the chain should be monitored. Convergence diagnostics seems to be rarely discussed in the context of the models used here. It should be noted that the sampling schemes discussed here have empirically shown to work well in practice. Overviews of convergence assessment methods are given in Cowles and Carlin (1996) and Robert and Casella (2004, pp. 459-510).

3.3 Model Diagnostics and Comparison

Bayesian methods for model diagnostics and assessment are an active and unsettled area of research. Most methods are based on assessing prediction quality, either by directly evaluating point or probabilistic prediction, or in terms of the predictive distribution

$$\int p(\boldsymbol{t}|\boldsymbol{\theta})f(\boldsymbol{\theta}|\boldsymbol{D})\,d\boldsymbol{\theta} \tag{3.4}$$

(Gelman et al. 2013). The first approach is harder to implement for failure time data; for censored observations predicted failure times can not be directly compared to an observed value. In addition, for models based on the Cox model, obtaining draws from the predictive distribution can be difficult. Usually,

$$p(\boldsymbol{t}|\boldsymbol{\theta}) = \prod_{i=1}^{n} p(t_i|\boldsymbol{\theta},\boldsymbol{z}_i)$$

in equation 3.4 is a probability density function. For failure time data, $p(t_i|\boldsymbol{\theta},\boldsymbol{z}_i)$ is given for discrete failure time data analyzed via failure indicators by

$$\prod_{i=1}^{t_i} p(y_{it}=1|\boldsymbol{\theta},\boldsymbol{z}_{it})^{y_{it}}(1-p(y_{it}=0|\boldsymbol{\theta},\boldsymbol{z}_{it}))^{y_{it}},$$

for continuous failure time by

$$p(t_i|\boldsymbol{\theta},z_i) = \begin{cases} G(t_i|\boldsymbol{\theta},z_i)h(t_i|\boldsymbol{\theta},z_i)^{\nu_i} & \text{if } t_i \text{ is not interval censored} \\ G(l_i|\boldsymbol{\theta},z_i) - G(r_i|\boldsymbol{\theta},z_i) & \text{else.} \end{cases}$$

For some criterions proper priors are necessary. These methods can not be used as Bayesian P-splines are based on improper priors. For failure time analysis, if there is qualitative knowledge about the failure process, this can be used for model assessment by inspecting the shape of the hazard. An overview over methods for failure time data is presented in this section.

3.3.1 Criterion Based Methods

A criterion based on prediction quality is the L-measure, embedded in the framework of minimizing posterior predictive loss developed by Gelfand and Ghosh (1998). The L-measure by Ibrahim et al. (2001a) uses a decomposition in prediction variance and a bias term weighted by $0 < u < 1$:

$$L^{\star}(\boldsymbol{t},u) = \sum_{i=1}^{n} Var(g(t_i)_{rep}|y_i) + u\sum_{i=1}^{n}(g(t_i) - \mu_i)^2, \tag{3.5}$$

where $(t_i)_{rep}$ denotes replications of failure times. The function $g(\cdot)$ is usually taken as $\log(\cdot)$ for failure times are usually heavily skewed, and $\mu_i = E[g(t_{rep,i})|t_i]$. For censored data, 3.5 is replaced by 3.6, here $\boldsymbol{l}$ and $\boldsymbol{r}$ are censoring times.

$$L_{obs}(\boldsymbol{t},u) = \int\int_{\boldsymbol{l}}^{\boldsymbol{r}} L_2(\boldsymbol{t},u) f(g(\boldsymbol{t}_{cens})|\boldsymbol{\theta}) f(\boldsymbol{\theta}|\mathscr{D})\, dg(\boldsymbol{t}_{cens})\, d\boldsymbol{\theta}, \tag{3.6}$$

The L-measure can be estimated from MCMC output via:

$$\hat{L}_{obs}(\boldsymbol{t},u) = \sum_{i=1}^{n}\{\frac{1}{S}\sum_{j=1}^{S}(E[(g(t_{rep,j}))^2|\theta_j] - \hat{\mu}_i^2)\} + u\{\sum_{\{i:y_i obs\}}(\hat{\mu}_i - g(t_i))^2 +$$
$$\frac{1}{S}\sum_{j=1}^{S}[\sum_{\{i:t_i cens\}}(\mu_i - g(t_{rep,is}))^2].$$

$E[(g(t_{rep,j}))$ and $E[(g(t_{rep,j}))^2$ are often not available in closed form for failure time data, they can be replaced by their respective average obtained from a MCMC run. The criterion can be used to compare arbitrary models under right and interval censoring, as long as draws from the posterior predictive distribution can be obtained. Several methods for obtaining random deviates from failure time random variables using hazard rates are given by Devroye (1986, pp. 260–285). The simplest method is based on inverting the cumulative hazard. If $H(t)$ can be inverted, a draw from $f(t) = h(t)\exp(-H(t))$ can be obtained by $H^{-1}(e)$, where e is a draw from a standard exponential distribution with cdf $1-\exp(-t)$;

$$P(H^{-1}(e) \leq t) = P(e \leq H(t)) = 1 - \exp(-H(t)) = F(t).$$

This can also be used for to sample from $f(t|t > l)$ as necessary for the estimation of the L-measure in case of right censoring, in this case the hazard is given by

$$h(t|t > l) = f(t|t > l)/G(t|t > l) = \frac{f(t)I[t > l]}{G(l)} / \frac{G(t)}{G(l)} = \frac{f(t)I[t > l]}{G(t)}$$

and $H(t|t > l)$ is $\int_0^t h(t|t > l)$. For interval censoring the conditional survivor function $G(t|t > l, t < r)$ can be inverted. If H^{-1} is not available in closed form, a numerical solution can be used. In general obtaining draws from the predictive distribution is not always easy or feasible, especially for some nonparametric models considered here where the log-baseline is modeled via P-splines. Apart from this difficulty the criterion suffers from the disadvantage of using the data twice for estimation and model evaluation; every data point influences its own prediction positively, which can lead to an overestimation of prediction accuracy (Hastie et al. 2009, p. 228). Crossvalidation based criterions, measuring out-of-sample prediction accuracy avoid this.

The pseudomarginal likelihood (LPMPL) (Geisser and Eddy 1979) is often used for failure time modeling, it is defined as:

$$LPML = \sum_{i=1}^{n} \log(CPO_i),$$

where CPO_i is the *conditional predictive ordinate*

$$CPO_i = \int p(t_i|\boldsymbol{\theta},z_i)f(\boldsymbol{\theta}|\mathscr{D}_{-i})\,d\boldsymbol{\theta}$$

for individual i, where $\mathscr{D}_{-i}$ denotes the data excluding individual i. The CPO_i is usually estimated by a sample from a single MCMC run. A simple estimator is (Gelfand 1996):

$$\widehat{CPO}_i = \left[\frac{1}{S}\sum_{i=1}^{n}\frac{1}{p(t_i|\boldsymbol{\theta}^{(s)})}\right]^{-1}, \tag{3.7}$$

where $\boldsymbol{\theta}^{(s)}$ denotes draw s of the MCMC run. The estimator 3.7 can be unstable for low values of $p(t_i|\boldsymbol{\theta}^{(s)})$, alternative estimators using importance sampling have been proposed (Vehtari and Ojanen 2012), although the estimator has been found to work well in practice by Hanson (2006). It can be shown that asymptotically the pseudomarginal likelihood contains a penalty term for the number of parameters similar to the AIC (Gelfand and Dey 1994).

For Bayesian models, a penalty term is necessary that accounts for what is estimated from the data and how much information is provided by the prior. The deviance information criterion (DIC), proposed by Spiegelhalter et al. (2002),contains such a penalty term. It is defined as

$$DIC = DEV(\hat{\boldsymbol{\theta}}) + p_D \tag{3.8}$$

where $DEV(\hat{\boldsymbol{\theta}}) = -2\log p(\boldsymbol{t}|\hat{\boldsymbol{\theta}})$ is the deviance at $\hat{\boldsymbol{\theta}}$, measuring goodness of fit and the penalty term is

$$p_D = E_{f(\boldsymbol{\theta}|\mathscr{D})}[DEV] - DEV(\hat{\boldsymbol{\theta}}).$$

A simple estimate for the penalty term is

$$\hat{p}_D = \frac{1}{S}\sum_{s=1}^{S} DEV(\boldsymbol{\theta}_s) - DEV(\hat{\boldsymbol{\theta}}), \tag{3.9}$$

plugging 3.9 into 3.8 yields an estimator for the DIC, so that the DIC is very easy to compute via MCMC output. Under strong prior information $\hat{p}_D$ is much less than the absolute number of parameters. The likelihood used in failure time modeling is not a joint density, Banerjee and Carlin (2004) argue that under random, noninformative censoring the likelihood is still appropriate for Kullback-Leitner divergence on which the DIC is based.

3.3.2 Martingale Residuals

Several types of residuals have been proposed for failure time analysis. Useful for right-censored data are martingale residuals (MR) which can be derived from an alternative representation of the likelihood in terms of a stochastic process called counting process. Counting process theory is not necessary for this thesis but some rudimentary concepts are necessary to properly introduce martingale residuals. Following Therneau and Grambsch (2000), a counting process $N_i(t)$ at time t gives the number of failures of individuals i in the interval [0,t]. For nonrecurrent events $N_i(t)$ is either one or zero. $Y_i(t) = 1[i \in R(t)]$ is the at-risk process of individual i, indicating membership in the risk set at time t. An individuals counting process $N_i(t_i)$ can be decomposed into the sum of two processes:

$$N_i(t_i) = A_i(t_i) + M_i(t_i),$$

$$A_i(t_i) = \begin{cases} \int_0^{t_i} Y_i(u)h_i(u)du & \text{if } T_i \text{ is continous} \\ \sum_{l=1}^{t_i} Y_i(l)h_i(l) & \text{if } T_i \text{ is discrete.} \end{cases}$$

$M_i(t)$ is a martingale:

$$E[M_i(t_i)|F_s] = M_i(s),$$

where F_s is (informally) the data available at time s. The estimated residual process at time t is $N_i(x) - \hat{A}_i(x)$, the martingale residual $\hat{M}_i$ is estimated by

$$\hat{M}_i(\infty) = v_i - \hat{A}_i(t_i),$$

where v_i is the censoring indicator. The value of $\hat{M}_i(\infty)$ represents the difference between observed and expected number of events for individual i. Martingale residuals have properties that are similar to residuals from linear regression: Under the true model, they have expectation zero and are uncorrelated. Often the residuals are used to determine the functional form of a covariate by plotting it against the covariate, but they can also be used to directly compare models, e.g. Kneib and Hennerfeind (2008) use kernel densities of estimated martingale residuals at selected points in time to detect patterns of low predictive performance.

3.4 Bayesian P-Splines

3.4.1 Basic Concepts

In this section Bayesian smoothing via penalized splines (P-splines) is introduced by the example of linear regression with normally distributed errors. This section is based on Fahrmeir et al. (2013, pp. 413–452), more formal introductions can be found in Dierckx (2006) or Boor (2001). The Gibbs sampler given in this section can (with slight adjustments) directly be used for the probit model in the context of discrete time, and the lognormal for continuous time. Regression models using P-splines have the structure

$$y = f(\boldsymbol{x}) + \boldsymbol{e}, \tag{3.10}$$

where $\boldsymbol{e} \sim N(\boldsymbol{0}, \sigma^2 \boldsymbol{I})$. Interest lies in the function f, which is assumed to be an unknown smooth function of the continuous covariate x. The idea of spline-smoothing is to approximate f by a polynomial spline of degree l ≥ 0, with knot sequence $x_{min} = k_1 < k_2, .. < k_m = x_{max}$ spread in the domain of x. A function f is called a polynomial spline of degree h if it satisfies the following conditions:

1. f is $(l-1)$ times continuous differentiable
2. f is a polynomial of degree l in every interval $[k_j, k_{j+1})$ determined by the knots

A spline is a function consisting of local polynomials joined together at the knots satisfying smoothness restrictions guaranteeing overall smoothness of the spline.

For the special case $l = 0$ there are no smoothness requirements for f. The overall smoothness is determined by the degree l, while flexibility is controlled by number and placement of the knots. Every polynomial spline can be written as a weighted sum of u=l+m-1 basis functions, which define the polynomial spline:

$$f(x) = \sum_{i=1}^{u} B_i(x)\zeta_i.$$

Given fixed basis functions, estimation can proceed as for classical linear regression (with a large number of coefficients), where the parameters to be estimated are given by $\zeta_i, i = 1, \ldots u$. Probably best known is truncated power series basis (TP basis):

$$B_1(x) = 1,\ B_2(x) = z, \ldots, B_{l+1}(x) = z^l, \tag{3.11}$$

$$B_{l+2}(x) = (z-k_2)^l I[z > k_2], \ldots, B_{l+m-1} = (z-k_{m-1})^l I[z > k_{m-1}]. \tag{3.12}$$

Here, the design-matrix $\boldsymbol{B}(\boldsymbol{x})$ for the regression model 3.10 has the form:

$$\begin{bmatrix} 1 & x_1 & x_1^2 & \ldots & x_1^l & (z_1-k_2)^l I[z_1 > k_2] & \ldots & (z_1-k_{m-1})^l I[z_1 > k_{m-1}] \\ 1 & x_2 & x_2^2 & \ldots & x_2^l & (z_2-k_2)^l I[z_2 > k_2] & \ldots & (z_2-k_{m-1})^l I[z_2 > k_{m-1}] \\ \vdots & \vdots & \vdots & & \vdots & \vdots & & \vdots \\ 1 & x_n & x_n^2 & \ldots & x_n^l & (z_n-k_2)^l I[z_n > k_2] & \ldots & (z_n-k_{m-1})^l I[z_n > k_{m-1}] \end{bmatrix}.$$

In general, the design matrix $\boldsymbol{B}$ consists of evaluations of the basis functions, so that $\boldsymbol{B}_{ij}$ gives the value of the jth basis function, evaluated at the covariate value x_i.

Given an estimate for $\boldsymbol{\zeta}$, for example the least squares estimate $(\boldsymbol{B}^\top \boldsymbol{B})^{-1}\boldsymbol{B}^\top \mathbf{y}$, the function value $f(\cdot)$ at covariate value x_i is estimated by

$$\widehat{f(x_i)} = \underbrace{x_i^0\zeta_1 + \ldots + x_i^l\zeta_{l+1}}_{\text{term 1}} +$$

$$\underbrace{(x_i-k_2)^l I[x_i > k_2]\zeta_{l+2} + \ldots + (x_i-k_{m-1})^l I[z > k_{m-1}]\zeta_{l+m-1}}_{\text{term 2}}$$

and the estimated function can be plotted by evaluation of $\widehat{f}$ at a large number of points in the domain of x and interpolating between the function evaluations. Term 1 one can be understood as a global polynomial from which there are random deviations represented by term 2. Bayesian inference for the TPS basis functions proceeds by treating it like a mixed model, $\zeta_1, \ldots, \zeta_{l+1}$ being viewed as fixed effects, $\zeta_{l+2}, \ldots, \zeta_{l+m-1}$ being viewed as random effects. The TPS basis is intuitive, but numerically unstable; as the basis functions are unbounded they can become numerically imprecise for large covariate values. Additionally, basis functions become almost linear dependent for knots that are close to each other. A better alternative is given by B-spline basis functions (see figure 3.1), given by:

$$
\begin{aligned}
B_j^0(x) &= I(k_j \leq x < k_{j+1}), j = 1, \ldots, u-1 \\
B_j^1(x) &= \frac{x - k_{j-1}}{k_j - k_{j-1}} I(k_{j-1} \leq x < k_j) + \frac{k_{j+1} - x}{k_{j+1} - k_j} I(k_j \leq x < k_{j+1}) \\
&\vdots \\
B_j^l(x) &= \frac{x - k_{j-l}}{k_j - k_{j-l}} B_{j-1}^{l-1}(x) + \frac{k_{j+1} - x}{k_{j+1} - k_{j+1-l}} B_j^{l-1}(x).
\end{aligned}
$$

Due to the recursive definition, the inner knot sequence $k_1 < \ldots < k_m$, must be expanded to $k_{1-l} < \ldots < k_{m+l}$. For equidistant knots, the knots are found by

$$k_j = min(x) + (j-1) * s, j = 1 - l, \ldots, m + l,$$

with interval width $s = (\max(x) - \min(x))/(m-1)$. Here, knots are always taken as equidistant knots for reasons that will be made clear in the following. B-spline functions exhibit the following properties from which their numerical stability follows:

- **Nonnegativity:**
  $B(y) \geq 0$, for all y and every degree l.
- **Local definition:**
  B-splines basis function are at maximum positive in an interval spanned by l+2 knots. Every basis function overlaps with 2l basis functions.

- **Normalization:**
  It holds that $\sum_{i=1}^{u} B_j(x_i) = 1$, for every $x_i \in [\min(\boldsymbol{x}), \max(\boldsymbol{x})]$. This implies that an intercept is implicitly included in the design matrix.

- **Bounded range:**
  B-spline basis functions are bounded from above.

Although B-splines have superior numerical properties compared to the TPS basis, they define exactly the same set of functions for a given knot sequence (Fahrmeir and Kneib 2011, p. 38).

B-Spline basis functions can be derived as normalized differences of TPS basis functions. For equidistant knots, the formula is (Eilers and Marx 2010):

$$B_j^l(x) = (-1)^{l+1} \Delta^{d+1} B_{j,TPS}^l(x)/(s^l l!),$$

where s is the distance between knots and Δ^d is the difference operator of order d, defined by:

$$\begin{aligned}\Delta^1 \zeta_i &= \zeta_i - \zeta_{i-1}\\ \Delta^d \zeta_i &= \Delta^{d-1} \zeta_i - \Delta^{d-1} \zeta_{i-1}.\end{aligned}$$

To avoid overfitting, the flexibility of the fit is usually restricted. For frequentist estimation based on least squares, this is achieved by adding a quadratic penalty term to the least squares criterion:

$$c(\lambda) = (\boldsymbol{y} - \boldsymbol{B}\boldsymbol{\zeta})^\top (\boldsymbol{y} - \boldsymbol{B}\boldsymbol{\zeta}) + \lambda \boldsymbol{\zeta}^\top \boldsymbol{K} \boldsymbol{\zeta},$$

where $\lambda \in [0, \infty)$ is a weight term controlling smoothness of the fit and $\mathbf{K}$ is a penalty matrix, penalizing rough function estimates. The influence of λ is visualized in figure 3.3. O'Sullivan (1986) uses the integrated second derivative of the fitted curve as penalty term,

$$p(\lambda) = \lambda \int_{min(x)}^{max(x)} \{\sum_{i=1}^{n} f''(x_i)\}^2 du, \tag{3.13}$$

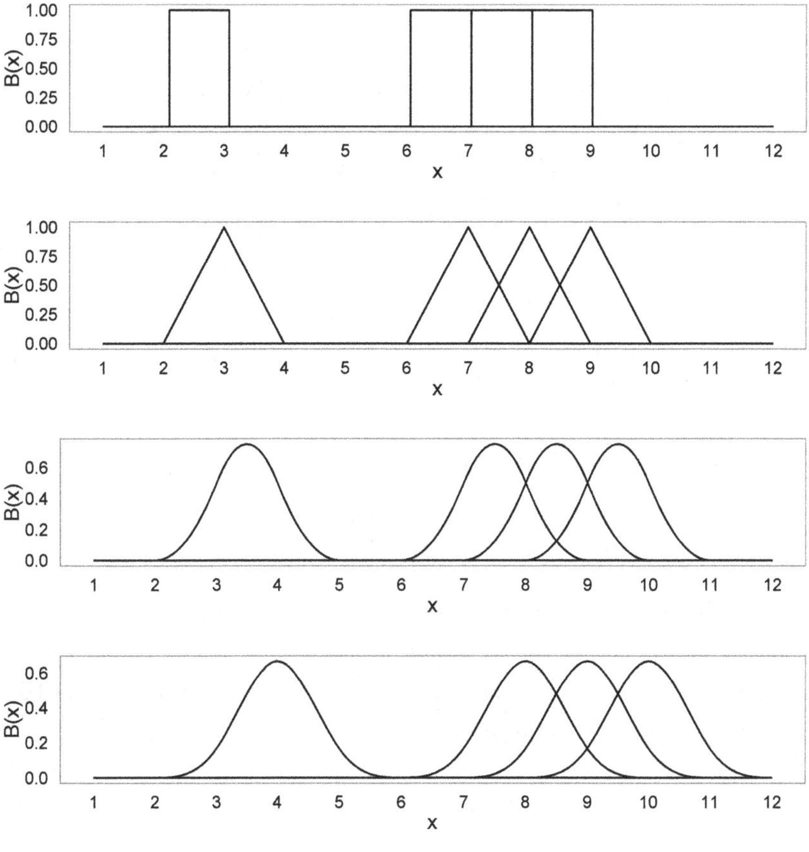

Figure 3.1: B-Spline basis functions of degree 0,1,2,3.

which can be taken as a measure for the curvature of a function. The penalty 3.13 can be written as $\boldsymbol{\zeta}^\top \boldsymbol{K} \boldsymbol{\zeta}$ with a penalty matrix $\boldsymbol{K}$ where

$$\boldsymbol{K}_{ij} = \int_{min(x)}^{max(x)} B_i''(u) B_j''(u)\, du.$$

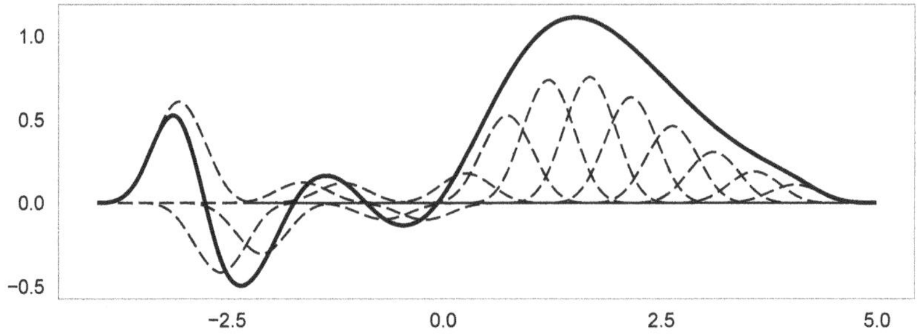

Figure 3.2: Function estimation via B-splines. The thick curve is the estimated function, given by the sum of scaled basis functions depicted in black.

The minimizer of 3.13 is $(\boldsymbol{B}^\top \boldsymbol{B} + \lambda \boldsymbol{K})^{-1} \boldsymbol{B}^\top \boldsymbol{y}$, which under the model

$$\boldsymbol{y} = f(\boldsymbol{x}) + \boldsymbol{\varepsilon} = \boldsymbol{B}(\boldsymbol{x})\boldsymbol{\zeta} + \boldsymbol{\varepsilon}$$

is clearly biased due to the penalty term. In terms of mean squared error this is generally compensated by the reduction of variance. A minimizer of 3.13 can be analytically found, even if the criterion is not represented in terms of basis functions but is instead represented as

$$(\boldsymbol{y} - f(\boldsymbol{x}))^T (\boldsymbol{y} - f(\boldsymbol{x})) + p(\lambda). \tag{3.14}$$

The minimizer of 3.14 is given by a spline having knots at every unique covariate value of x, called *smoothing spline* with basis functions very similar to B-Spline basis functions. Smoothing splines have in general excellent properties, they are implemented in a Bayesian framework by Hastie and Tibshirani (2000). Due to the high dimension of the design matrix, computational burden is very high. A compromise is used by Eilers and Marx (1996), where a penalty is based on the derivative of the estimated function. The first derivative of $f(x)$ for the B-Spline basis is given by

$$\sum_{j=1}^{u} B_j^{l'}(x)\zeta_i = -s^{-1} \sum_{j=1}^{u} \Delta\zeta_{j+1} B_j^{l-1}(x),$$

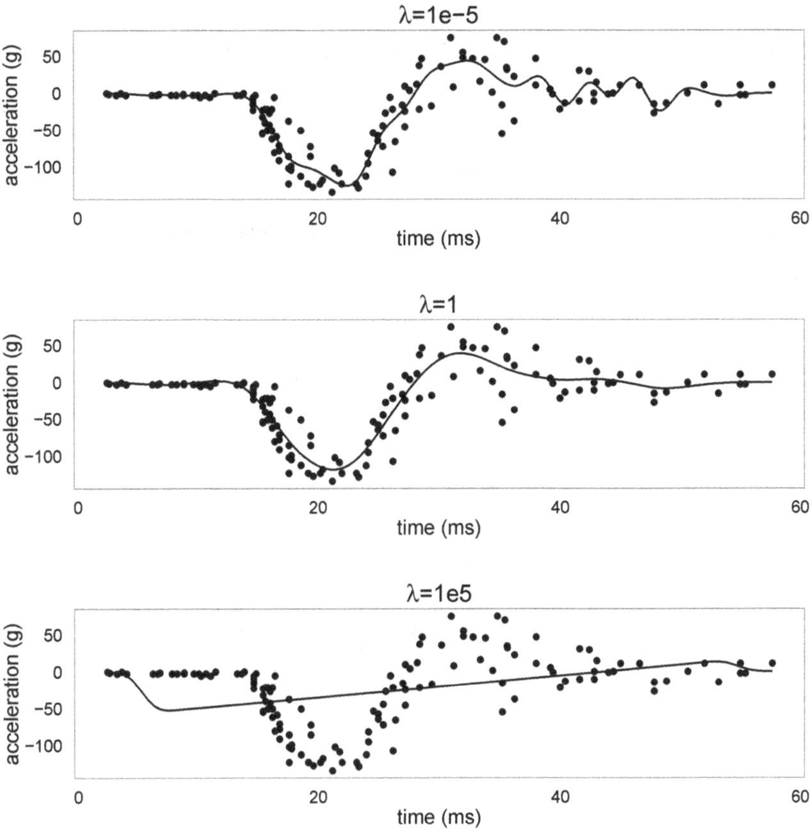

Figure 3.3: Influence of smoothing parameter. The first choice of λ leads to over- the third to underfitting. Used is the mcycle data set from R package MASS (Venables and Ripley 2002) on simulated motorcycle accidents. X-axis is time after impact, Y-axis is acceleration in g.

where s is the distance between the knots. In general it can be shown that the dth derivative depends on the dth order difference of neighbouring parameters. The summed squared difference of order d of adjacent coefficients approximates the integrated square of the dth derivative. This leads to the penalty:

$$\sum_{i=1}^{u}(\Delta^d \zeta_i)^2 = \boldsymbol{\zeta}^\top \boldsymbol{D}_d^\top \boldsymbol{D}_d \boldsymbol{\zeta} = \boldsymbol{\zeta}^\top \boldsymbol{K}_d \boldsymbol{\zeta}, \tag{3.15}$$

where $\boldsymbol{D}_t$ is a difference matrix, indexed by the order of the difference used, and $\boldsymbol{K}_t = \boldsymbol{D}_t^\top \boldsymbol{D}_t$. This combination of basis function and penalty is usually referred to as P-splines. In analogy to the scalar case, the difference matrices are recursively defined:

$$\boldsymbol{D}_t = \boldsymbol{D}_1 \boldsymbol{D}_{t-1}$$

For instance, the relevant quantities of 3.15 for a difference penalty of order 2 are given by:

$$\boldsymbol{D}_2 = \begin{bmatrix} 1 & -1 & & & \\ & 1 & -1 & & \\ & & \ddots & \ddots & \\ & & & 1 & -1 \end{bmatrix} \begin{bmatrix} 1 & -1 & & & \\ & 1 & -1 & & \\ & & \ddots & \ddots & \\ & & & 1 & -1 \end{bmatrix} =$$

$$\begin{bmatrix} 1 & -2 & 1 & & \\ & 1 & -2 & 1 & \\ & \ddots & \ddots & \ddots & \\ & & 1 & -2 & 1 \end{bmatrix}, \boldsymbol{D}_2 \boldsymbol{\zeta} = \begin{bmatrix} \zeta_3 - 2\zeta_2 + \zeta_1 \\ \vdots \\ \zeta_K - 2\zeta_{K-1} + \zeta_{K-2} \end{bmatrix},$$

,

$$\boldsymbol{K}_2 = \begin{bmatrix} 1 & -2 & 1 & & & & & & \\ -2 & 5 & -4 & 1 & & & & & \\ 1 & -4 & 6 & -4 & 1 & & & & \\ & & \ddots & \ddots & \ddots & & & & \\ & & & & 1 & -4 & 6 & -4 & 1 \\ & & & & & 1 & -4 & 5 & -2 \\ & & & & & & 1 & -2 & 1 \end{bmatrix}.$$

Compared to smoothing splines, the dimension of $\boldsymbol{\zeta}$ has been reduced from the number of unique values of x to $u = l + m - 1$, depending on the choice of l and the number of knots m. A general strategy to choose m is to use a large enough number of knots so that the data would be overfit without the penalty, for example m=30.

For equidistant knots, this strategy gives good results in sparse-data situations, as the estimated function interpolates better as with unequally spaced knots, while in regions there would hardly be any gain in precision using a larger number of knots (Eilers and Marx 2010). As such, the simple choice of equdistant knots gives good results. For nonequdistant knots the penalty matrix $\boldsymbol{K} = \boldsymbol{D}^\top \boldsymbol{D}$ can be adjusted to include weights via $\boldsymbol{K} = \boldsymbol{D}^\top \boldsymbol{W}\boldsymbol{D}$.

To transfer the difference penalty 3.15 to a Bayesian framework, the difference penalty can be interpreted as prior knowledge regarding the smoothness of the function $f(\cdot)$. A smoothness prior for $\boldsymbol{\zeta}$ has been developed by Lang and Brezger (2004) in the form of the random walk priors. The difference penalty of order d translates to a random walk of order d of the regression coefficient:

$$\zeta_k = \Delta^d \zeta_k + u_k,$$

with $u_k \sim N(0, \xi^2)$ and diffuse priors $\propto c$ for $\zeta_1, \ldots \zeta_d$. e.g. for a random walk of order 1 and 2:

$$\zeta_k = \zeta_{k-1} + u_k, \; \zeta_k = 2\zeta_{k-1} - \zeta_{k-2} + u_k.$$

This prior can be written as:

$$\boldsymbol{\zeta} | \xi^2 \propto \left(\frac{1}{\xi^2}\right)^{\mathrm{rank}(\boldsymbol{K})/2} \exp\left(-\frac{1}{2\xi^2} \boldsymbol{\zeta}^\top \boldsymbol{K} \boldsymbol{\zeta}\right) \tag{3.16}$$

The prior 3.16 is improper as a result of the diffuse prior for the initial values. It has $\mathrm{rank}(\boldsymbol{K}) = k - d$. All columns and rows of the penalty matrix $\mathbf{K}$ add up to $\mathbf{0}$. It can be shown that the nullspace of the penalty matrix is spanned by global polynomial of order d-1, which therefore is not penalized (Kneib 2006, p. 36). The global variance parameter ξ^2 controls the smoothness of the fit. For $\lim \xi^2 \to 0$, no deviations from the global polynomial would be allowed, for a difference penalty of order 2, a straight line would be obtained. For $\lim \xi^2 \to \infty$, the function estimate would become extremly rough and would fit the data at hand extremly well. As prior knowledge about ξ^2 is usually rare, ξ^2 is assigned a hyperprior, so the smoothing parameter is estimated from the data. A conditional conjugate inverse gamma hyperprior $\xi^2 \sim IG(a_0^\xi, b_0^\xi)$ is normally used. Very low hyperparameters a_0^ξ, b_0^ξ, e.g. 0.001 for both are usually chosen. A diffuse prior for the variance parameter would result in a improper posterior. For unknown σ^2, the prior $\sigma^2 \sim IG(a_0^\sigma, b_0^\sigma)$ is a convenient choice as it is conditionally conjugate. Under the Gaussian likelihood the resulting full conditionals are all conjugate. A Gibbs sampler for the model parameters of 3.10 alternates between sampling from the conditional distributions of the regression coefficients, the smoothing variance, and the residual variance. The full conditional of $\boldsymbol{\zeta}$ is

$$N(\frac{1}{\sigma^2}\boldsymbol{B}^\top\boldsymbol{B}+\frac{1}{\xi^2}\boldsymbol{K})^{-1}\frac{1}{\sigma^2}\boldsymbol{B}^\top\boldsymbol{y},(\frac{1}{\sigma^2}\boldsymbol{B}^\top\boldsymbol{B}+\frac{1}{\xi^2}\boldsymbol{K})^{-1}). \tag{3.17}$$

The full conditional distributions for σ^2 and ξ^2 are both $IG(\cdot,\cdot)$, with parameters

$$a_0^\sigma + n/2, b_0^\sigma + \boldsymbol{\varepsilon}^\top\boldsymbol{\varepsilon}/2$$

for the residual variance, and

$$a_0^\xi + \text{rank}(\boldsymbol{K})/2, b_0^\xi + \boldsymbol{\zeta}^\top\boldsymbol{K}\boldsymbol{\zeta}/2$$

for the smoothing variance. The computation of the moments of 3.17 can be done very quickly: Due to the local definition of the B-splines, the design matrix $\boldsymbol{B}$ is sparse and the precision matrix $\boldsymbol{\Sigma}_\zeta^{-1} = \frac{1}{\sigma^2}\boldsymbol{B}^\top\ \boldsymbol{B} + \frac{1}{\xi^2}\boldsymbol{K}$ is a band matrix with bandwidth $\max(d,l)$ where h is the degree of the spline and d is the order of the random walk. Specialized algorithms can be used to quickly invert $\boldsymbol{\Sigma}_\zeta^{-1}$ which is highly relevant for an iterative algorithm such as the Gibbs sampler. In the following section, extensions from univariate smoothing are introduced.

3.4.2 Extended Linear Predictor

The model 3.10 can be written in terms of the *linear predictor* as:

$$\begin{aligned}\boldsymbol{y} &= \boldsymbol{\eta} + \boldsymbol{\varepsilon}\\ \boldsymbol{\eta} &= \boldsymbol{B}\boldsymbol{\zeta}.\end{aligned}$$

Extensions of the model can be represented in terms of extensions of the linear predictor. Following Fahrmeir et al. (2013, p. 183) the linear predictor including all effects can generically be written as

$$\boldsymbol{\eta} = \boldsymbol{Z\beta} + \boldsymbol{W\alpha} + f_1(\boldsymbol{x}_1) + \ldots + f_r(\boldsymbol{x}_r) =$$

$$\boldsymbol{Z\beta} + \boldsymbol{W\alpha} + \boldsymbol{B}_1\boldsymbol{\zeta}_1 + \ldots.\boldsymbol{B}_r\boldsymbol{\zeta}_r. \tag{3.18}$$

where $\boldsymbol{Z\beta}$ are fixed effects, $\boldsymbol{W} = bdiag(\boldsymbol{W}_1,...,\boldsymbol{W}_p)$ is the design matrix corresponding to random effects $\boldsymbol{\alpha} = (\boldsymbol{\alpha}_1^\top,...,\boldsymbol{\alpha}_p^\top)^\top$, $\boldsymbol{B}_i\boldsymbol{\zeta}_i, i = 1,...,m$ are effects represented via basis functions, B-spline or other. Description of estimation techniques is easier and conciser via this representation. The extensions will be discussed in detail in the following.

3.4.2.1 Fixed and Random Effects

For Bayesian inference all parameter are taken as random variables so that the distinction between fixed and random effects is somewhat misleading, as these labels are common in the literature they are nonetheless used here.

For fixed effects $\boldsymbol{Z\beta}$, the prior distributions $\boldsymbol{\beta} \sim N(\boldsymbol{t},\boldsymbol{T})$ and diffuse priors $\boldsymbol{\beta} \propto$ *constant* are common. $\boldsymbol{Z}$ is the usual design matrix for fixed effects. The full conditional is multivariate normal with variance

$$\boldsymbol{\Sigma}_{\boldsymbol{\beta}} = \sigma^2(\boldsymbol{Z}^\top\boldsymbol{Z} + \sigma^2\boldsymbol{T}^{-1})^{-1}$$

and expectation

$$\boldsymbol{\mu}_{\boldsymbol{\beta}} = \boldsymbol{\Sigma}_{\boldsymbol{\beta}}/\sigma^2(\boldsymbol{Z}^\top[\boldsymbol{y} - \boldsymbol{\eta} + \boldsymbol{Z\beta}] + \sigma^2\boldsymbol{T}^{-1}\boldsymbol{t}),$$

(Fahrmeir and Kneib 2011, p. 213). The case $\boldsymbol{T}^{-1} = \boldsymbol{0}$ corresponds to a diffuse prior. To account for cluster-specific heterogenity, Gaussian random effects can be included in the model. These can also be brought into the basis function framework by viewing e.g. a random intercept α_i as function of a index variable $x_j^\star$, taking values 1,...,p, so that $g(x_{ij}^\star) = \alpha_i$, see Brezger and Lang (2006), but the classical perspective is taken here.

For random effects, the prior $\boldsymbol{\alpha}_i \sim N(\mathbf{0},\boldsymbol{Q}), i=1,...,p$ can be used. An inverse Wishart hyperprior denoted by $IW(a_0,\boldsymbol{B}_0)$ for the covariance matrix $\boldsymbol{Q}$ is conditionally conjugate and allows within-cluster correlation of random effects, while random effects are indendent across clusters. Gyperparameters are a_0 and $\boldsymbol{B}$. The full conditonal distribution of random effects $\boldsymbol{\alpha}_i$ is of the exact same form as for fixed effects, the distribution is $N(\boldsymbol{\mu}_{\boldsymbol{\alpha}_i},\boldsymbol{\Sigma}_{\boldsymbol{\alpha}_i})$ where

$$\boldsymbol{\Sigma}_{\boldsymbol{\alpha}_i} = \sigma^2(\boldsymbol{W}_i^\top \boldsymbol{W}_i + \sigma^2 \boldsymbol{Q}^{-1})^{-1}$$

and

$$\boldsymbol{\mu}_{\boldsymbol{\alpha}_i} = \boldsymbol{\Sigma}_{\boldsymbol{\alpha}_i}/\sigma^2(\boldsymbol{Z}_i^\top [\boldsymbol{y}_i - \boldsymbol{\eta}_i + \boldsymbol{W}_i\boldsymbol{\alpha}_i] + \sigma^2 \boldsymbol{Q}^{-1}).$$

The vector $\boldsymbol{\alpha}$ could also be updated in one large block, but this is not necessary as random effects are conditionally independent across individuals (Gamerman 1997). The full conditional distribution of $\boldsymbol{Q}$ is $IW(a^\star,\boldsymbol{B}^\star)$, where

$$a^\star = a_0 + p/2, \quad \boldsymbol{B}^\star = \boldsymbol{B}_0 + \frac{1}{2}\sum_{i=1}^{p} \boldsymbol{\alpha}_i \boldsymbol{\alpha}_i^\top.$$

As an alternative, $\boldsymbol{Q}$ can be taken as $\text{diag}(\upsilon_1,...,\upsilon_q)$. Using the prior

$$\upsilon_i \sim IG(a_0^{\alpha_i}, b_0^{\alpha_i}),$$

the full conditionals are

$$\upsilon_i \sim IG(a_0^{\alpha_i} + p/2, b_0^{\alpha_i} + \frac{1}{2}\sum_{i=1}^{n} \alpha_{ij}^2)),$$

for j=1,...p, where α_{ij} is the jth element of α_i. There are parallels between random effects and P-spline coefficients. It can be shown that for a model

$$\boldsymbol{y} = \boldsymbol{B}(\boldsymbol{x})\boldsymbol{\zeta} \tag{3.19}$$

with a prior of the form $f(\boldsymbol{\zeta}|\xi^2) \propto \exp\{-\frac{1}{2\xi^2}\boldsymbol{\zeta}\boldsymbol{K}\boldsymbol{\zeta}\}$, where $\boldsymbol{K}$ is rank deficient, and

$\boldsymbol{B}(\boldsymbol{x})$ is matrix of B-spline basis functions, the model 3.19 can be written as mixed model

$$\boldsymbol{y} = \boldsymbol{U}\boldsymbol{\gamma} + \boldsymbol{G}\boldsymbol{\upsilon},$$

where $\boldsymbol{\gamma}$ are fixed and $\boldsymbol{\upsilon}$ are random effects. For the B-Spline basis, the random effects $\boldsymbol{\upsilon}$ represent deviations from a global polynomial described by $\boldsymbol{U}\boldsymbol{\gamma}$, in complete analogy to the TPS-basis. It follows that $\text{var}(\boldsymbol{y}|\boldsymbol{U}\boldsymbol{\gamma})$ is not a diagonal matrix, so that B-splines marginally induce correlation (Fahrmeir and Kneib 2011, p. 230). For Gaussian $\boldsymbol{y}$, $cov(y_i, y_j|\boldsymbol{U}\boldsymbol{\gamma})$ can be given in closed form, in general the correlation is a function of the closeness of covariate values x_i, x_j.

The marginal and conditional hazard usually differ under the presence of random effects, as do the marginal and conditional hazard, so that parameter interpretation differs. This is a specialized topic for failure time analysis and this point will not be stressed in this thesis, in general the implementation of random effects, in this context called frailties will be mentioned and implicitly a conditional perspective is taken.

3.4.2.2 Multiple Functions $f_1(\boldsymbol{x}_1) + ... + f_r(\boldsymbol{x}_r)$

Models with linear predictor containing several functions $f_1, ... f_r$ have an idenfication problem: As the linear predictor

$$\boldsymbol{\eta}^\star = f_1(\boldsymbol{x}_1)^\star + ... f_r(\boldsymbol{x}_r)^\star, \text{ with } f_1(\boldsymbol{x}_1)^\star = f_1(\boldsymbol{x}_1) + c,\ f_2(\boldsymbol{x}_2)^\star + c = f_2(\boldsymbol{x}_2) - c$$

equals the linear predictor

$$\boldsymbol{\eta} = f_1(\boldsymbol{x}_1) + ... + f_r(\boldsymbol{x}_r),$$

the mean level of the functions $f_1(\boldsymbol{x}_1) + f_2(\boldsymbol{x}_2) +, ..., + f_r(\boldsymbol{x}_r)$ is not identified and identification constraints must be imposed. Using constraints of the form $\boldsymbol{C}_j\boldsymbol{\zeta}_j = \boldsymbol{0}$, the prior 3.16 can be adjusted to

$$\boldsymbol{\zeta}_j|\xi_j^2 \propto \left(\frac{1}{\xi_j^2}\right)^{\text{rank}(\boldsymbol{K}_j)/2} \exp\left(-\frac{1}{2\xi_j^2}\boldsymbol{\zeta}_j^\top \boldsymbol{K}\boldsymbol{\zeta}_j\right) I[\boldsymbol{C}_j\boldsymbol{\zeta}_j = 0], \text{ for } j = 1, ..., r, \quad (3.20)$$

(Lang et al. 2014). A natural choice is $\boldsymbol{C}_j = \boldsymbol{B}_j(x_j)$ so that

$$\sum_{i=1}^{n} \hat{f}_1(x_{1i}) = \sum_{i=1}^{n} \hat{f}_2(x_{2i}) = ... = \sum_{i=1}^{n} \hat{f}_r(x_{ri}) = 0. \tag{3.21}$$

Here, the functions $f_j(\cdot), j = 1,..,r$ represent deviations from the global mean set by the intercept $\boldsymbol{\beta}_0$ which is always assumed to be included. For the normal likelihood, the conditional distribution of $\boldsymbol{\zeta}_j$ is still normal with moments 3.22, constrained to $\boldsymbol{C}_j\boldsymbol{\zeta}_j = \boldsymbol{0}$. In general, draws from

$$\boldsymbol{x}|\boldsymbol{\mu},\boldsymbol{Q}^{-1} \propto \exp(-\frac{1}{2}\left(\boldsymbol{x}-\boldsymbol{\mu})^\top \boldsymbol{Q}(\boldsymbol{x}-\boldsymbol{\mu})\right) I[\boldsymbol{Ax}=\boldsymbol{0}],$$

can be generated by the following steps (Rue and Held 2005, pp. 37–39):

1. Sample $\boldsymbol{x}^\star$ from $N(\boldsymbol{\mu},\boldsymbol{Q}^{-1})$.
2. Compute $\boldsymbol{x} = \boldsymbol{x}^\star - \boldsymbol{Q}^{-1}\boldsymbol{A}^\top(\boldsymbol{AQ}^{-1}\boldsymbol{A}^\top)^{-1}\boldsymbol{Ax}$.

For the restriction 3.21, step 2 can be done quickly as $\boldsymbol{A} = \boldsymbol{1}^\top\boldsymbol{B}_i$ is a row vector. Another, perhaps less elegant approach, is to center the functions in every iteration of the Gibbs sampler. The mean of each function subsequently is added to the intercept so that the posterior is unchanged. The full conditional of all regression coefficientes corresponding to basis function matrices $\boldsymbol{B}_j(\boldsymbol{x}_j)$ is given by:

$$\boldsymbol{\Sigma}_j = (\frac{1}{\sigma^2}\boldsymbol{B}_j^\top\boldsymbol{B}_j + \frac{1}{\xi_j^2}\boldsymbol{K}_j)^{-1}, \boldsymbol{\mu}_j = \boldsymbol{\Sigma}_j\frac{1}{\sigma_j^2}\boldsymbol{B}_j^\top[\boldsymbol{y} - \boldsymbol{\eta} + \boldsymbol{B}_j(\boldsymbol{x}_j)\boldsymbol{\zeta}_j], \tag{3.22}$$

(Lang and Brezger 2004). The full conditional distribution of ξ_j^2 is

$$\xi_j^2 \sim IG(a_0^{\xi_j} + \frac{\text{rank}(\boldsymbol{K}_j)}{2}, b_0^{\xi_j} + \frac{1}{2}\boldsymbol{\zeta}_j^\top\boldsymbol{K}_j\boldsymbol{\zeta}_j).$$

Some further extensions useful for failure time analysis can be included by varying the elements of $\boldsymbol{B}_j$ and $\boldsymbol{K}_j$ which are given in the following.

Varying Coefficients

Varying coefficients have the form

$$z_1\boldsymbol{\beta}_1(\boldsymbol{x}_1)+\ldots+z_k\boldsymbol{\beta}_k(\boldsymbol{x}_k)$$

(Hastie and Tibshirani 1993). Interaction between the covariates z_j and x_j are modeled by allowing the effect of the *interaction variable* to z_j vary over the domain of the *effect modifier* x_j. Conditional on the effect modifier, the effect is linear. This can be estimated in the given framework by defining the matrix of basis functions

$$diag(z_j)\boldsymbol{B}_j^{\star}(x_j)=\boldsymbol{B}_j,$$

where $\boldsymbol{B}^{\star}$ is the usual matrix of B-splines basis functions. The most interesting effect modifier for failure time analysis is time, allowing time varying effects. Often the interaction variables are binary variables, defining nonlinear deviations for subgroups.

Seasonal Effect and Time Trends

Suppose that historical time is observed as 1,2,...,N, with period length g. A flexible formulation that allows for time-varying seasonal effects assumes, (Kneib 2006, pp. 39–40):

$$\zeta_{\text{seas},i}=-(\zeta_{\text{seas},1}+\ldots+\zeta_{\text{seas},g-1})\sim N(0,\xi^2_{\text{seas}}).$$

This can be written as

$$\boldsymbol{\zeta}_{\text{seas}}|\xi^2_{\text{seas}}\propto\exp(-\frac{1}{2\xi^2_{\text{seas}}}\boldsymbol{\zeta}^{\top}_{\text{seas}}\boldsymbol{K}_{\text{seas}}\zeta_{\text{seas}}),$$

by defining

$$\boldsymbol{D}_{\text{season}}=\begin{bmatrix}1 & \ldots & 1 & & \\ & \ddots & \ldots & \ddots & \\ & & 1 & \ldots & 1\end{bmatrix},$$

$\boldsymbol{K}_{\text{season}} = \boldsymbol{D}_{\text{season}}^{\top}\boldsymbol{D}_{\text{season}}$, where $\boldsymbol{D}_{\text{season}}$ has dimension $(N-g)\times N$ and the entry 1 is repeated g times in every row of $\boldsymbol{D}_{\text{season}}$. The rank of $\boldsymbol{K}_{\text{season}}$ is given by N-g+1. The parameter ξ^2_{seas} controls the variation of the seasonal effects over time. For $\lim \xi^2_{\text{seas}} \to 0$, the seasonal effects become constant over time. The corresponding design matrix $\boldsymbol{B}_{\text{seas}}$ is a matrix of binary indicators. It is also possible to include time trends, to this end historical time can be treated exactly like a time-varying covariate.

3.4.2.3 Sampling Scheme

The sampling scheme for the normal model is given by sampling scheme 1. At every step the most recent values of all conditioning parameters are used. As can be seen the steps for random effects, fixed effects and regression coefficients for P-splines respectively basis function coefficients are very similar to each other. In general the main estimation problem will lie in determining regression coefficients.

3.4.2.4 Alternative Priors for Variance Parameter

The inverse gamma prior for the smoothing and random effect variance is a convenient choice due to its conjugacy to the normal distribution, but the distribution exhibits some undesirable properties (Polson and Scott 2011), (Gelman 2006): (1) For small samples the hyperparameter for the variance parameter can have large influence on estimates, making it a bad choice if the prior is supposed to be non-informative. (2) The distribution is biased against zero. For random effects and P-spline coefficients this corresponds to completely linear effects and the absence of heterogenity, both situations are important to detect. As an alternative, the use of the Cauchy distribution truncated from below at zero, with pdf

$$f(\sigma|d) \propto (1+\sigma^2/d)^{-(d+1)/2}$$

called half-cauchy distribution, has been advocated by Gustafson (1997) for the variance parameter and by Gelman (2006) for the standard deviation. A half-

Sampling scheme 1

1 Draw fixed effects from $N(\boldsymbol{\mu}_{\beta}, \boldsymbol{\Sigma}_{\beta})$ where

$$\boldsymbol{\Sigma}_{\beta} = \sigma^2(\mathbf{Z}^\top \mathbf{Z} + \sigma^2 \boldsymbol{T}^{-1})^{-1}, \text{ and}$$

$$\boldsymbol{\mu}_{\beta} = \frac{1}{\sigma^2}\boldsymbol{\Sigma}_{\beta}(\mathbf{Z}^\top[\mathrm{y} - \boldsymbol{\eta} + \boldsymbol{Z\beta}] + \sigma^2 \boldsymbol{T}^{-1}\boldsymbol{t})$$

2 For j=1,...,m: Draw regression coefficients for basis functions coefficients from $N(\boldsymbol{\mu}_{\zeta_j}, \boldsymbol{\Sigma}_{\zeta_j})$ where

$$\boldsymbol{\Sigma}_{\zeta_j} = (\frac{1}{\sigma^2}\boldsymbol{B}_j^\top \boldsymbol{B}_j + \frac{1}{\xi_j^2}\boldsymbol{K}_j)^{-1}, \boldsymbol{\mu}_{\zeta_j} = \boldsymbol{\Sigma}_{\zeta_j}\frac{1}{\sigma^2}\boldsymbol{B}_j^\top[\mathrm{y} - \boldsymbol{\eta} + \boldsymbol{B}_j(\boldsymbol{x}_j)\boldsymbol{\zeta}_j],$$

correct the samples by the steps given in section 3.4.2.2

3 For i=1,...,p: Draw random effects from $N(\boldsymbol{\mu}_{\alpha_i}, \boldsymbol{\Sigma}_{\alpha_i})$ with

$$\boldsymbol{\Sigma}_{\alpha_i} = \sigma^2(\boldsymbol{W}_i^\top \boldsymbol{W}_i + \sigma^2 \boldsymbol{Q}^{-1})^{-1} \text{ and}$$

$$\boldsymbol{\mu}_{\alpha_i} = \frac{1}{\sigma^2}\boldsymbol{\Sigma}_{\alpha_i}(\boldsymbol{Z}_i^\top[\mathrm{y}_i - \boldsymbol{\eta}_i + \boldsymbol{W}_i\boldsymbol{\alpha}_i] + \sigma^2 \boldsymbol{Q}^{-1})$$

4 For i=1,...,r: Draw smoothing variance from $IG(a_0^{\xi_i} + \frac{\mathrm{rank}(\boldsymbol{K}_i)}{2}, b_0^{\xi_i} + \frac{1}{2}\boldsymbol{\zeta}_i^\top \boldsymbol{K}_i \boldsymbol{\zeta}_i)$

5 Draw σ^2 from $IG(a_0^{\sigma} + \frac{n}{2}, b_0^{\sigma} + \frac{\boldsymbol{\varepsilon}^\top \boldsymbol{\varepsilon}}{2})$

6 Draw $\boldsymbol{Q}$ from $IW(a_0 + p/2, \frac{1}{2}\sum_{i=1}^{p} \boldsymbol{\alpha}_i \boldsymbol{\alpha}_i^\top)$, or for nondiagional $\boldsymbol{Q}$:
For j=1,...p: Draw var(α_i) from $IG(a_0^{\alpha_i} + p/2, b_0^{\alpha_i} + \frac{1}{2}\sum_{i=1}^{n} \alpha_{ij}^2))$

cauchy prior with d=1 for a standard deviation corresponds to an inverted-beta distribution $\propto (\sigma^2)^{(b-1)}(1+\sigma^2)^{-(a+b)}$ with parameters a=b=$1/2$ for the variance (Polson and Scott 2011). For some highly variable functions a global variance parameter can be inappropriate. Variable function estimates can be obtained by letting the variance vary across coefficients. This can for example be done by introducing gamma distributed weights, leading to a marginal t-distribution (Lang and Brezger 2004). In general the inverse gamma prior is used as default choice here.

3.4.2.5 Extrapolation

If there is interest in predicting a function beyond the boundaries of the data set, say for a point $x^\star > \max(\boldsymbol{x}_j)$, samples for the necessary regression coefficients $\zeta_{j,u+1}, \zeta_{j,u+2}...$ are obtained by continuing the random walk of order d of the regression coefficents $\boldsymbol{\zeta}$. Equidistant knots are added to the knots sequence and the corresponding basis functions have to be computed. For example for a difference penalty or order one, draws for $\zeta_{j,u+1}$ are obtained from $N(\zeta_u^s, \xi^{2(s)})$, for s=1,...,S. The function value at $x^\star$ can be estimated by

$$\hat{f}(x^\star) = \frac{1}{S}\sum_{i=1}^{S}\sum_{k=1}^{u^\star} B_{jk}(x^\star)$$

(Brezger and Lang 2006), where $u^\star$ is the number of columns of B_{jk} after adding enough knots so that $\sum_{k=1}^{u^\star} B_{jk} = 1$.

4 Discrete Time Models

As noted in section 2.3, by the introduction of failure indicators $y_{ij}, i = 1, ..., n, j = 1, ..., t_i$ a Bernoulli likelihood is obtained and estimation can proceed as for binary regression - allowing that time can be treated like an arbitrary covariate whose effect can be smoothed. This is not the case for continuous time models. The linear predictor for discrete time models has the generic form

$$\boldsymbol{\eta} = \boldsymbol{\eta} + \boldsymbol{Z\beta} + \boldsymbol{W\alpha} + \boldsymbol{B}_1(\boldsymbol{x}_1) + ... + \boldsymbol{B}_m(\boldsymbol{x}_m),$$

where for this chapter it is always assumed that $\boldsymbol{x}_1 = \boldsymbol{t}$, so that $\boldsymbol{B}_1(\boldsymbol{t})$ describes the baseline hazard. The basis function matrices are allowed to have the forms given in section 3.4.1 and may further depend on process time.

This chapter is structured as follows: At first the generalized linear model framework is given, embedded in which iteratively weighted least squares (IWLS) proposals can be derived which can be used for continuous time models as well. Some important models for discrete time are discussed. Subsequently estimation based on data augmentation scheme is discussed.

The baseline hazard is estimated unified via P-splines for all discrete time models. The simplest specification is a constant baseline hazard in every period t, using P-splines of order 0 where the columns of $\boldsymbol{B}(\boldsymbol{t})$ are given by binary indicators. The difference penalty suppresses large jumps in sparse data settings where estimation is unstable. By design, these occur towards the end of the observation time for failure time data. Splines of higher order can be used as well to obtain smoother estimates, allowing the baseline hazard to vary within intervals.

4.1 Estimation Based on GLM Methodology

Following McCulloch and Searle (2001, pp. 135–143) the Bernoulli distribution belongs to the exponential family of distributions, which can be analyzed in the generalized linear model framework. Distributions in the exponential family can be written as

$$f(y_i|\theta,\phi) = \exp\{(y\theta_i - b(\theta_i))/\phi + c(y_i,\phi)\}, \tag{4.1}$$

where θ and ϕ are referred to as the natural and the scale parameter and $b(\cdot)$ and $c(\cdot)$ are functions specific to the distribution. The expectation and variance depend on the natural parameter:

$$E[y_i] = \mu_i = b'(\theta),$$

$$\text{var}(y_i) = b''(\theta) = \phi v(\mu_i).$$

For regression analysis, μ_i is related to the linear predictor η_i by the link function

$$\eta = g(\mu_i),$$

with inverse $r(\eta_i) = \mu_i$. The Bernoulli with pmf

$$p_i^{y_i}(1-p_i)^{1-y_i}$$

has natural parameter $\theta_i = \log(p_i/1-p_i)$, the pmf written in the form 4.1 is:

$$f(y_i|\theta) = \exp(y_i\theta_i - \log(1+\exp(\theta_i))),$$

where $b(\theta_i) = \log(1+\exp(\theta_i))$, $\phi = 1$ and $c(y,\phi) = 0$, so $b'(\theta) = EY_i = p_i$ and $\text{var}(y_i) = b''(\theta_i) = p_i(1-p_i)$. IWLS proposals will be used here for the Bernoulli and the Poisson likelihood, both of which have $\phi = 1$, so with no loss of generality $\phi = 1$ is taken hereafter.

Suppose the model only includes fixed effects, so that the linear predictor η_i is given by $\boldsymbol{z}_i^\top \boldsymbol{\beta}$. The full conditional of $\boldsymbol{\beta}$ is in general not conditional conjugate for GLMs and a Metropolis-Hastings update can be used. For maximum likelihood estimation, maximizing the loglikelihood

$$L(\boldsymbol{\beta}) = \sum_{i=1}^{n} (y_i\theta_i - \log(1+\exp(\theta_i)))$$

with respect to $\boldsymbol{\beta}$ usually can not be done analytically. Iterative numerical methods can be used, using local information about the surface of the loglikelihood to find the maximum. This information is valuable in finding a proposal distribution. Fisher scoring computes the maximum via the following iteration rule:

$$\boldsymbol{\beta}^{(s+1)} = \boldsymbol{\beta}^{(s)} + \boldsymbol{I}(\boldsymbol{\beta}^{(s)})^{-1} s(\boldsymbol{\beta}), \tag{4.2}$$

where $s(\boldsymbol{\beta})$ is the score vector and $\boldsymbol{I}(\boldsymbol{\beta}^{(s)})$ is the Fisher information at $\boldsymbol{\beta}$. It can be shown that the Fisher information and the score vector for exponential family distributions can always be written as

$$\boldsymbol{I}(\boldsymbol{\beta}^{(s)}) = \mathbf{Z}^\top \mathbf{W}\mathbf{Z}, \text{ and} \tag{4.3}$$

$$s(\boldsymbol{\beta}) = \sum_{i=1}^{n} (y_i - \mu_i) w_i g'(\mu_i) z_i^\top = \mathbf{Z}^\top \mathbf{W}\boldsymbol{\Delta}(\mathbf{y} - \boldsymbol{\mu}), \tag{4.4}$$

where $\mathbf{W} = \text{diag}(w_1, \ldots w_n)$, $w_i = [v(\mu_i)(g'(\mu_i))^2]^{-1}$ and $\boldsymbol{\Delta} = \text{diag}(g'(\mu_1), \ldots g'(\mu_n))$ depend on $\boldsymbol{\beta}^{(s)}$. For canonical link functions it holds that $\theta = \eta$ and $g'(\mu_i) = 1/\text{var}(\mu_i)$, hence the expressions for the diagonal of W are simplified. Plugging the expressions 4.3 and 4.4 into 4.2, this can be viewed as a weighted least square regression

$$\boldsymbol{\beta}^{(k+1)} = (\mathbf{Z}^\top \mathbf{W}\mathbf{Z})^{-1} \mathbf{Z}^\top \mathbf{W} \dot{\mathbf{y}}(\boldsymbol{\eta}^{(k)}),$$

of working observations

$$\dot{\mathbf{y}}(\boldsymbol{\eta}^{(k)}) = \boldsymbol{\eta}^{(k)} + \boldsymbol{\Delta}(\boldsymbol{\eta}^{(k)})[\mathbf{y} - \boldsymbol{\mu}(\boldsymbol{\eta}^{(k)})],$$

on $\mathbf{Z}$, as $\text{var}(\dot{\mathbf{y}}) = \mathbf{W}^{-1}$. This estimator also would be obtained under the working model

$$\dot{\mathbf{y}}(\hat{\boldsymbol{\eta}}^{(k)}) \sim N(\mathbf{Z}^\top \boldsymbol{\beta}, \mathbf{W}^{-1}). \tag{4.5}$$

The idea behind IWLS proposals by Gamerman (1997) is to approximate the full conditional distribution of $\boldsymbol{\beta}$

$$\propto \exp(\log(f(\boldsymbol{y}|\boldsymbol{\theta})) + \log(f(\boldsymbol{\theta})))$$

by replacing the likelihood $f(\boldsymbol{y}|\boldsymbol{\theta})$ by the likelihood corresponding to the model 4.5, hence approximating the likelihood by a Gaussian likelihood obtained via one Fisher scoring step. Under a prior distribution

$$\propto \exp(-\frac{1}{2}(\boldsymbol{\beta} - \boldsymbol{t})^\top \boldsymbol{T}^{-1}(\boldsymbol{\beta} - \boldsymbol{t})),$$

where $T^{-1} = \mathbf{0}$ represents a diffuse prior $\boldsymbol{\beta} \propto const$, this gives

$$\propto \exp(-\frac{1}{2}\left((\dot{\boldsymbol{y}} - \boldsymbol{Z}\top\boldsymbol{\beta})^\top [\mathbf{Z}^\top \mathbf{W}\mathbf{Z}]^{-1}(\dot{\boldsymbol{y}} - \boldsymbol{Z}^\top\boldsymbol{\beta}) + (\boldsymbol{\beta} - \boldsymbol{t})^\top \boldsymbol{T}^{-1}(\boldsymbol{\beta} - \boldsymbol{t})\right)),$$

as proposal distribution. This is proportional to a normal distribution with covariance matrix and expectation:

$$\begin{aligned}\boldsymbol{\Sigma}_{\boldsymbol{\beta}}(\boldsymbol{\eta}^{(s)}) &= (\mathbf{Z}^\top \mathbf{W}\mathbf{Z} + \boldsymbol{T}^{-1})^{-1}\\ \boldsymbol{m}_{\boldsymbol{\beta}}(\boldsymbol{\eta}^{(s)}) &= \boldsymbol{\Sigma}_{\boldsymbol{\beta}}(\boldsymbol{\eta}^{(s)})(\mathbf{Z}^\top \boldsymbol{W}\dot{\boldsymbol{y}} + \boldsymbol{T}^{-1}\boldsymbol{t}),\end{aligned}$$

where $\boldsymbol{W} = \boldsymbol{W}(\boldsymbol{\eta}^{(s)})$ and $\dot{\boldsymbol{y}} = \dot{\boldsymbol{y}}(\boldsymbol{\eta}^{(s)})$. The extension to the full predictor

$$\boldsymbol{\eta} + \boldsymbol{Z}\boldsymbol{\beta} + \boldsymbol{W}\boldsymbol{\alpha} + \boldsymbol{B}_1(\boldsymbol{x}_1) + \ldots + \boldsymbol{B}_r(\boldsymbol{x}_r)$$

is straightforward. To update $\boldsymbol{\zeta}_j$, with corresponding penalty matrix $\boldsymbol{K}_j/\xi^{2(s-1)}$ at iteration s, the mean of the proposal is changed to the mean obtained under the working model $\dot{\boldsymbol{y}} \sim N(\boldsymbol{\eta}, \boldsymbol{W}^{-1})$, which is:

$$\boldsymbol{m}_{\boldsymbol{\zeta}_j}(\boldsymbol{\eta}^{(s)}) = \boldsymbol{\Sigma}_{\boldsymbol{\zeta}_j}(\boldsymbol{\eta}^{(s)})(\mathbf{Z}^\top \boldsymbol{W}[\dot{\boldsymbol{y}} - \boldsymbol{\eta}^{(s)} + \boldsymbol{B}_j\boldsymbol{\zeta}_j^{(s)}]), \tag{4.6}$$

with covariance matrix

$$\mathbf{\Sigma}_{\zeta_j}(\boldsymbol{\eta}^{(s)}) = [\mathbf{Z}^\top \mathbf{W}\mathbf{Z} + \mathbf{K}_j/\xi^{2(s-1)}]^{-1}, \tag{4.7}$$

where the weights and working observations are evaluated at $\boldsymbol{\eta}^{(s)}$,

$$\begin{aligned}\boldsymbol{\eta}^{(s)} =& \mathbf{Z}\boldsymbol{\beta}^{(s)} + \mathbf{W}\boldsymbol{\alpha}^{(s)} + \mathbf{B}_1\boldsymbol{\zeta}_1^{(s)} + ... + \mathbf{B}_{j-1}\boldsymbol{\zeta}_{j-1}^{(s)} + \\ & \mathbf{B}_j\boldsymbol{\zeta}_j^{(s-1)} + \mathbf{B}_{j+1}\boldsymbol{\zeta}_{j+1}^{(s-1)} + ... + \mathbf{B}_r\boldsymbol{\zeta}_r^{(s-1)}.\end{aligned}$$

This has the form of a regression on partial residuals $\dot{\mathbf{y}}(\boldsymbol{\eta}^{(s)}) - \boldsymbol{\eta}^{(s)} + \mathbf{B}_j\boldsymbol{\zeta}_j^{(s)}$. To update $\boldsymbol{\zeta}^{(s)}$ at iteration s, a proposal $\boldsymbol{\beta}^\star$ from a multivariate normal distribution with covariance and expectation 4.6 is drawn and and accepted with probability

$$\alpha(\boldsymbol{\zeta}^{(s)}, \boldsymbol{\zeta}^\star) = \min\left(\frac{L(\mathbf{y}|\boldsymbol{\zeta}^\star) f(\boldsymbol{\zeta}^\star|(\xi_i^2)^{(s-1)})\phi(\boldsymbol{\zeta}^{(s)}|\mathbf{m}_{\zeta_j}(\boldsymbol{\eta}^\star), \mathbf{\Sigma}_{\zeta_j}(\boldsymbol{\eta}^\star))}{L(\mathbf{y}|\boldsymbol{\zeta}^{(s)}) f(\boldsymbol{\zeta}^{(s)}|(\xi_i^2)^{(s-1)})\phi(\boldsymbol{\zeta}^\star|\mathbf{m}_{\zeta_j}(\boldsymbol{\eta}^{(s)}), \mathbf{\Sigma}_{\zeta_j}(\boldsymbol{\eta}^{(s)}))}, 1\right). \tag{4.8}$$

where $\boldsymbol{\eta}^\star = \boldsymbol{\eta}^{(s)} + \mathbf{B}_j(\boldsymbol{\zeta}_j^\star - \boldsymbol{\zeta}_j^{(s)})$ and $\phi(\mathbf{x}|\mathbf{a}, \mathbf{B})$ denotes the density of the multivariate normal distribution with moments $\mathbf{a}, \mathbf{B}$ evaluated at $\mathbf{x}$. Implementing the identification restriction $\sum_{i=1}^n f(x) = 0$ is easier here by centering the functions in every iteration, as adjusting the proposal distribution to the conditional density $N(\mathbf{m}, \mathbf{\Sigma}|\mathbf{A}\boldsymbol{\zeta} = \mathbf{0})$ would involve evaluating furthermore normalizing constants due to the conditioning. Updating fixed and random effects is done in analogy, the only differences are that random effects $\boldsymbol{\alpha}_1, ..., \boldsymbol{\alpha}_n$ are updated seperately and the prior is fixed for fixed effects. This leads to sampling scheme 2 (Brezger and Lang 2006).

To evaluate $\alpha(\boldsymbol{\zeta}^{(s)}, \boldsymbol{\zeta}^\star)$, the moments $\mathbf{m}_{\zeta_j}(\boldsymbol{\eta}^\star)$ and $\mathbf{\Sigma}_{\zeta_j}(\boldsymbol{\eta}^\star)$ conditional on

$$\boldsymbol{\eta}^\star = \boldsymbol{\eta}^{(s)} + \mathbf{B}_j(\boldsymbol{\zeta}_j^\star - \boldsymbol{\zeta}_j^{(s)})$$

have to be computed. This is computationally costly as it involves calculation of $\mathbf{W}(\boldsymbol{\eta}^\star)$, $\mathbf{\Delta}(\boldsymbol{\eta}^\star)$, $\dot{\mathbf{y}}(\boldsymbol{\eta}^\star)$ and the inversion of $(\mathbf{Z}^\top \mathbf{W}(\boldsymbol{\eta}^\star)\mathbf{Z} + \mathbf{T}^{-1})$. Brezger and Lang (2006) give a modification of the proposal distribution. Here $\boldsymbol{\zeta}^{(s)}$ in the linear predictor is replaced by $\mathbf{m}_{\zeta_j}(\boldsymbol{\eta}^{(s-1)})$, the mean of the proposal distribu-

Sampling scheme 2
1 For i=1,...,m: Draw a proposal $\boldsymbol{\zeta}_j^\star$ from a normal distribution with expectation 4.7 and covariance 4.6, compute 4.8, set $\begin{cases} \boldsymbol{\zeta}_j^{(s)} = \boldsymbol{\zeta}_j^\star & \text{with probability } \alpha(\boldsymbol{\zeta}^{(s)},\boldsymbol{\zeta}^\star)) \\ \boldsymbol{\zeta}_j^{(s)} = \boldsymbol{\zeta}_j^{(s-1)} & \text{with probability } 1-\alpha(\boldsymbol{\zeta}^{(s)},\boldsymbol{\zeta}^\star)) \end{cases}$
2 For i=1,...,p: Draw random effects by steps analog to basis function coefficients
3 Draw fixed effects by steps analog to basis function coefficients
4 Draw smoothing variance by step 4, sampling scheme 1
5 Draw variance of random effects by step 6, sampling scheme 1

tion used at iteration $s-1$, in the calculation of the moments of the proposal distribution, independent if the proposal was accepted or not. Writing $\boldsymbol{\eta}_{\zeta_{j,m}}^{(s)} = \boldsymbol{\eta}^{(s)} + \boldsymbol{B}_j(\boldsymbol{m}_{\zeta_j}(\boldsymbol{\eta}^{(s-1)}) - \boldsymbol{\zeta}_j^{(s)})$, the moments of the proposal distribution for $\boldsymbol{B}_j\boldsymbol{\zeta}_j$ are given by

$$\boldsymbol{\Sigma}_{\zeta_j}(\boldsymbol{\eta}_{\zeta_{j,m}}^{(s)}) = (\mathbf{Z}^\top \boldsymbol{W}\mathbf{Z} + \boldsymbol{K}_j^{-1}/\xi^{2(s-1)})^{-1} \tag{4.9}$$

$$\boldsymbol{m}_{\zeta_j}(\boldsymbol{\eta}_{\zeta_{j,m}}^{(s)}) = \boldsymbol{\Sigma}_{\zeta_j}(\boldsymbol{\eta}_{\zeta_{j,m}}^{(s)})(\mathbf{Z}^\top \boldsymbol{W}[\dot{\boldsymbol{y}} - \boldsymbol{\eta}_{\zeta_{j,m}}^{(s)} + \boldsymbol{B}_j\boldsymbol{m}_{\zeta_j}(\boldsymbol{\eta}^{(s-1)})]), \tag{4.10}$$

with $\boldsymbol{W} = \boldsymbol{W}(\boldsymbol{\eta}_{\zeta_{j,m}}^{(s)})$ and $\dot{\boldsymbol{y}} = \dot{\boldsymbol{y}}(\boldsymbol{\eta}_{\zeta_{j,m}}^{(s)})$, so that the proposal distribution is independent from the current state $\boldsymbol{\zeta}^{(s)}$. Hence the moments of the proposal distribution have to be computed only once. In addition to reducing computation time, acceptance rates are often higher.

A draw is accepted with probability

$$\alpha(\boldsymbol{\zeta}^{(s)},\boldsymbol{\zeta}^\star) = \min(1, \frac{L(\boldsymbol{y}|\boldsymbol{\zeta}^\star) f(\boldsymbol{\zeta}^\star|\xi^{2(s-1)}) \phi(\boldsymbol{\zeta}^{(s)}|\boldsymbol{m}(\boldsymbol{\eta}_{\zeta_{j,m}}^{(s)}), \boldsymbol{\Sigma}_{\zeta_j}(\boldsymbol{\eta}_{\zeta_{j,m}}^{(s)}))}{L(\boldsymbol{y}|\boldsymbol{\zeta}^{(s)}) f(\boldsymbol{\zeta}^{(s)}|\xi^{2(s-1)}) \phi(\boldsymbol{\zeta}^\star|\boldsymbol{m}(\boldsymbol{\eta}_{\zeta_{j,m}}^{(s)}), \boldsymbol{\Sigma}_{\zeta_j}(\boldsymbol{\eta}_{\zeta_{j,m}}^{(s)})}. \tag{4.11}$$

Adjusting the proposal distribution to $N(\boldsymbol{a},\boldsymbol{B}|\boldsymbol{A}\boldsymbol{\zeta} = \mathbf{0})$ does not change the acceptance probability: We have

$$\phi(\boldsymbol{\zeta}^{\star}|\boldsymbol{m}_{\zeta_j},\boldsymbol{\Sigma}_{\zeta_j},\boldsymbol{A\zeta}^{\star}=0)=\frac{\phi(\boldsymbol{\zeta}^{\star}|\boldsymbol{m}_{\zeta_j},\boldsymbol{\Sigma}_{\zeta_j})f(\boldsymbol{Ax}|\boldsymbol{x})}{\phi(\boldsymbol{A\zeta}^{\star}|\boldsymbol{Am}_{\zeta_j},\boldsymbol{A\Sigma}_{\zeta_j}\boldsymbol{A}^{\top})}, \tag{4.12}$$

it can be shown (Rue and Held 2005, p. 38) that

$$\log f(\boldsymbol{Ax}|\boldsymbol{x})=-\frac{1}{2}\log|\boldsymbol{AA}^{\top}|. \tag{4.13}$$

As $\boldsymbol{A\zeta}^{\star}=\boldsymbol{A\zeta}^{(s)}=\boldsymbol{0}$, the only factor not canceling in 4.12 if plugged into 4.11 is $\phi(\boldsymbol{\zeta}^{\star}|\boldsymbol{m}_{\zeta_j},\boldsymbol{\Sigma}_{\zeta_j})$. The sampling scheme is given in the following.

Sampling scheme 3

1 For i=1,...,m:
Draw a proposal $\boldsymbol{\zeta}_j^{\star}$ from a normal distribution with expectation 4.10 and covariance 4.9, compute 4.11,

$$\text{set}\begin{cases}\boldsymbol{\zeta}_j^{(s)}=\boldsymbol{\zeta}_j^{\star} & \text{with probability } \alpha(\boldsymbol{\zeta}^{(s)},\boldsymbol{\zeta}^{\star}))\\ \boldsymbol{\zeta}_j^{(s)}=\boldsymbol{\zeta}_j^{(s-1)} & \text{with probability } 1-\alpha(\boldsymbol{\zeta}^{(s)},\boldsymbol{\zeta}^{\star}))\end{cases}$$

2 For i=1,...,p: Draw random effects by steps analog to basis function coefficients
3 Draw fixed effects by steps analog to basis function coefficients
4 Draw smoothing variance by step 4, sampling scheme 1
5 Draw variance of random effects by step 6, sampling scheme 1

Another adjustment is to compute the weight matrix only every kth iteration, or even keep it fixed, which usually does not impair convergence.

IWLS proposals allow fully automatic blockwise updates and usually have high acceptance rate. In terms of mixing better solutions are possible, for example a closer approximation of the full conditional distribution can be constructed. However the approach of IWLS proposals is quite general and the literature on the models this thesis deals with mainly uses this approach. The idea behind IWLS proposals was also used by Hennerfeind (2006) as blueprint for the development of proposal distributions for continuous time models which will be discussed in

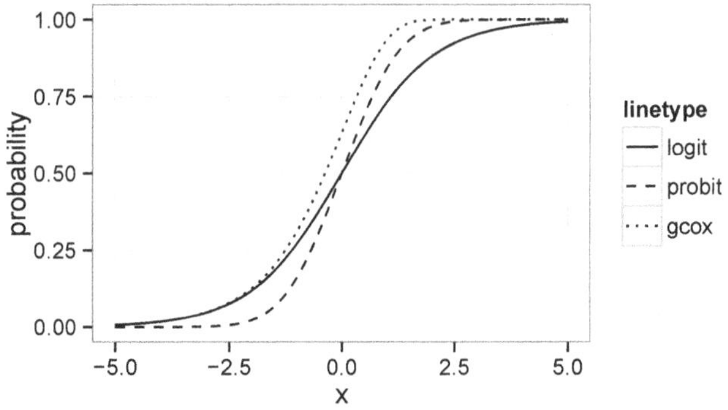

Figure 4.1: The most common response functions

section 6.3. As such, all models in this thesis can be estimated via adjustments of sampling schemes 1-3.

In the following sections, some important models corresponding to different choices of link functions are discussed.

4.1.1 Grouped Cox

The grouped Cox model is the discrete time analog to the Cox model in continuous time with hazard

$$h(t_i|\eta_i) = h_0(t_i)\exp(\eta_i) \tag{4.14}$$

(Kalbfleisch and Prentice 1973). Given an unobservable continuous random variable T*, the probability of failure in the interval $[a_{j-1}, a_j)$, given survival until a_{j-1}, under the Cox model with relative risk hazard $h_0(t_i)\exp(\eta_i)$, is given by:

$$= P(T^* \in [a_{j-1}, a_j)|\eta_{ij}, T^* > a_{j-1}) = 1 - \exp\{-\exp(\eta_{ij})\int_{a_{j-1}}^{a_j} h_0(u)\,du\}. \tag{4.15}$$

Equation 4.15 holds for covariates that are time-constant or constant in every interval $[a_{j-1}, a_j), j = 1, ..., m$. The notation η_{ij} denotes the linear predictor where the covariates are evaluated at a_{j-1}. Grouping T*, gives

$$P(T=t|\eta_{it}) = 1-\exp\{-\exp\{\overline{\eta}_{it}+\alpha_0(t)\}\},$$

where $\alpha_0(t) = \log\int_{t-1}^{t} h_0(u)du$ and $\overline{\eta}$ is the linear predictor without the baseline hazard and without time-varying effects. In a GLM context the corresponding link function $g(x) = \log(-\log(1-x))$ is referred to as complementary log-log link. As η is unchanged by the discretization of the time scale, regression coefficients and estimated effects can be directly interpreted in terms of T* (Fahrmeir and Tutz 2001, p. 140).

Independent of the connection to the relative risk model, the complementary log-log link provides a good fit for binary models if one of the categories is more frequent than the other, due to the asymmetry of the response function (Cameron and Trivedi 2005, p. 466). This holds obviously for most data sets for failure time. For IWLS proposals, the computation of

$$\boldsymbol{W}_{it} = [\exp(\eta_{it}-\exp(\eta_{it}))]^2/(h_{it}(1-h_{it}))$$

and

$$\boldsymbol{\Delta}_{it} = ([\exp(\eta_{it}-\exp(\eta_{it})]^{-1})$$

is necessary which can be unstable and slow. An alternative method will be given in section 4.2.3.

4.1.2 Logistic Model

Under the logistic model the hazard is given by

$$h(t_i|\eta_{ij}) = \frac{\exp(\eta_{ij})}{1+\exp(\eta_{ij})},$$

and covariates act multiplicatively on the conditional odds:

$$\frac{P(T=t|T\geq t)}{P(T>t|T\geq t)} = \exp(\eta_{it}). \tag{4.16}$$

The factor $\exp(\beta_k)$ can be interpreted as effect of an one unit change of covariate z_k in terms of the odds (given that the remaining covariates are held fixed). The working observations have the easy form

$$\eta_{it} + \frac{(y_{it} - \mu_{it})}{\mu_{it}(1 - \mu_{it})},$$

and the weights are given by $\mu_{it}(1 - \mu_{it})$, where

$$\mu_{it} = P(T = t | T \geq t) = \frac{\exp(\eta_{it})}{1 + \exp(\eta_{it})}. \tag{4.17}$$

For an underlying discretized variable $T^\star$, where δ is the interval width, 4.16 implies that in the limiting case $\lim \delta \to 0$ the hazard of the Cox model is recovered (Fleming and Harrington 1991, pp. 127–128).

The right side of 4.17 is the cdf of a logistic distribution, this distribution has similar shape to the normal distribution with slightly wider tails. The logit model gives results which are very similar to the probit model where the response function is given by the cdf of a standard normal distribution. For the latter model, a completion Gibbs sampler can be set up that bypasses the necessity for Metroplis-Hastings updates completely as all conditional distributions are fully conjugate (under the priors considered here). Such sampling schemes for various models are discussed in the following.

4.2 Estimation Based on Latent Variable Representation

4.2.1 Probit Model

A completion Gibbs sampler for the probit model was developed by Albert and Chib (1993). Let $\tilde{Y}_{it}, i = 1, \ldots, n$ be random variables, related to Y_{it} by:

$$Y_{it} = \begin{cases} 1 & \tilde{Y}_{it} > 0 \\ 0 & \tilde{Y}_{it} \leq 0 \end{cases}$$

so that $P(Y_{it}=1)=P(\tilde{Y}_{it}>0)$. Under the model

$$\tilde{\boldsymbol{Y}}_i=\boldsymbol{\eta}_i+\sigma\boldsymbol{\varepsilon}_i \tag{4.18}$$

where $\varepsilon_i \sim N(0,\boldsymbol{I})$, we have $\mathrm{P}(Y_{it}=1)=\Phi(\eta_{it}/\sigma)$. As

$$\Phi(\boldsymbol{\eta}^{\star}/\sigma^{\star})=\Phi(\boldsymbol{\eta}/\sigma),\forall c\neq 0,$$

where $\eta^{\star}=c\eta^{\star}$ and $\sigma^{\star}=\sigma c$, only the ratio η/σ is identified and σ is usually fixed at $\sigma=1$ (Greene 2012, p. 686). Due to the deterministic relationship between Y and $\tilde{\mathrm{Y}}$, $f(y_{it}|\eta_{it},\tilde{y}_{it})=1[\tilde{y}_{it}>0]$ and

$$\tilde{Y}_{it}\sim TN_{(0,\infty)}(\eta_{it},1),$$

where $TN_{(0,\infty)}(a,b)$ denotes a normal distribution, truncated to the interval $(0,\infty)$ with mean a and variance b.

Suppose again for introductory purposes there are only fixed effects so that $\eta_{it}=\boldsymbol{z}_{it}^{\top}\boldsymbol{\beta}$. The joint posterior distribution of $\tilde{\boldsymbol{Y}}=(\tilde{\boldsymbol{Y}}_1,...,\tilde{\boldsymbol{Y}}_n)^{\top}$ and $\boldsymbol{\beta}$ is

$$g(\tilde{\boldsymbol{Y}},\boldsymbol{\beta}|\mathscr{D})\propto f(\boldsymbol{\beta})\prod_{i=1}^{n}\prod_{j=1}^{t_i}(I[\tilde{Y}_{it}>0]I[y_{it}=1]+I[\tilde{Y}_{it}\leq 0]I[y_{it}=0])\phi(\tilde{Y}_{it}|\boldsymbol{z}_{ij}^{\top}\boldsymbol{\beta},1). \tag{4.19}$$

Integrating $\tilde{\boldsymbol{Y}}$ out of 4.19 gives the marginal distribution

$$\propto f(\boldsymbol{\beta})\prod_{i=1}^{n}\prod_{j=1}^{t_i}\Phi(\boldsymbol{z}_{it}^{\top}\boldsymbol{\beta})^{y_{it}}(1-\Phi(\boldsymbol{z}_{it}^{\top}\boldsymbol{\beta}))^{1-y_{it}}$$

so $g(\tilde{\boldsymbol{Y}},\boldsymbol{\beta}|\mathscr{D})$ is a completion of the posterior distribution $f(\boldsymbol{\beta}|\mathscr{D})$. The model is equivalent a Bernoulli GLM with response function $\Phi(x)=\int_{-\infty}^{x}\phi(u|0,1)\,du$. Sampling from truncated normal distributions can be quickly done, in Robert (1995) and Geweke (1991) efficient methods are given. As the necessity of Metropolis-Hastings steps is completely bypassed, sampling scheme 4 is computationally much cheaper than the use of IWLS proposals. The sampling scheme for the full linear predictor 3.18 is then given as:

Sampling scheme 4
1 For $i = 1,...,n, j = 1,...,t_i$: Draw $\tilde{y}_{ij}^{(s)}$ from $TN_{I_{ij}}(\eta_{ij},1)$, where $I_{ij} = \begin{cases} (0,\infty) & \text{if } y_{it} = 1 \\ (-\infty,0] & \text{if } y_{it} = 0 \end{cases}$
2 Draw parameter using sampling scheme 1, with σ fixed at 1

4.2.2 Scale Mixtures of Normals

The family of scale mixtures of normal distributions consists of distributions that can be represented as $\int f(Y\lambda|\lambda)h(\lambda)\,d\lambda$, where $Y \sim N(0,1)$ and $\lambda > 0$ (Andrews and Mallows 1974). Some useful scale mixtures are given in table 4.1. Conditional on λ, Y is distributed as $N(0,\lambda^2)$. If g is a scale mixture, $f(Y|\lambda)h(\lambda)$ is by definition a completion of $g(\cdot)$. This leads to the representation

$$\tilde{y}_{it} = \eta_{it} + \varepsilon_{it}, \quad \varepsilon_{it}|\lambda_{it} \sim N(0,\lambda_{it}),$$

for distributions from the scale mixture family. Sampling scheme 4 for the probit model can be extended by an additional block for $\boldsymbol{\lambda}$ (Albert and Chib 1993). The conditional distributions are adjusted to account for the scale factor but conditional conjugacy is preserved: The conditional distribution of e.g. fixed effects with prior $N(\boldsymbol{\beta}_0,\boldsymbol{B}_0)$ is

$$N((\boldsymbol{Z}^\top \boldsymbol{W}\boldsymbol{Z})^{-1}[\boldsymbol{Z}^\top \boldsymbol{W}(\tilde{\boldsymbol{y}} - \boldsymbol{\eta} + \boldsymbol{Z}\boldsymbol{\beta}) + \boldsymbol{B}_0^{-1}\boldsymbol{\beta}_0]),$$

where $W = \text{diag}(\boldsymbol{\lambda}_1^{-1},...,\boldsymbol{\lambda}_n^{-1})$. In general the moments of the conditional distribution are the same with the exception of the additional weight matrix $\boldsymbol{W}$. An important choice is $\lambda_{it} \sim IG(\omega/2,\omega/2)$, resulting in a marginal t-distribution with ω degrees of freedom. The parameter a can be estimated from the data, it is usually updated via a Metropolis-Hastings step, but is often kept fixed at a low value. The t-link is a robust alternative to more common link functions, as it can be shown to be less influenced by outliers. In addition, as $F_7^t(x/1.5484) \approx F_{logistic}(x)$, where

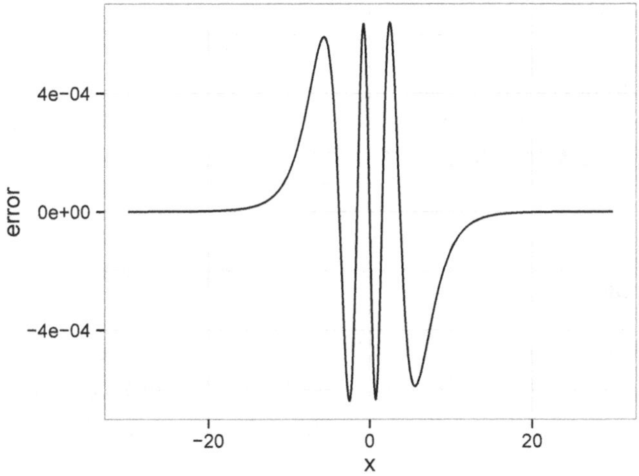

Figure 4.2: $F_7^t(x/1.5484) - F^{\text{logistic}}(x)$

$F_\nu^t(x)$ denotes the cdf of a t-distributed variable with ω degrees of freedom, the logistic model can be very well approximated via the t model (Liu 2004), see figure 4.2. For the t-link, the distribution $h(\lambda_{it}|\cdot)$ is available in closed form and given by

$$\lambda_{it} \sim IG(\frac{\omega+1}{2}, \frac{2}{\omega+(\tilde{y}_{it}-\eta_{it})^2}).$$

An exact solution is available as well as the logistic distribution belongs to the scale mixture family, but sampling λ is difficult for this model as λ follows a Kolmogorov-Smirnov distribution for which the cdf and pdf are only available in an infinite series representation (Devroye 1986, p. 161).

Table 4.1: Some mixtures

Marginal distribution of e_it	Mixture component λ_i
Student-t(v)	$\lambda_i \sim IG(\nu/2, \nu/2)$
Laplace(J)	$\lambda_i \sim \text{Exp}(0.5J)$
Standard logistic	$\lambda_i = (2K)^2, K \sim$ Kolmogoro-Smirnov

Sampling scheme 5: Scale Mixtures
1 For $i = 1,...,n, j = 1,...,t_i$: Draw λ_{it} from $f(\lambda_{it}\mid\cdot)$
2 Draw parameters and latent data as for sampling scheme 4, with additional weight matrix $\mathbf{W}$=diag$(\boldsymbol{\lambda}_1^{-1},...,\boldsymbol{\lambda}_n^{-1})$

4.2.3 Grouped Cox II

For the grouped Cox model with link function $\log(-\log(1-\mu_{it}))$ we have $P(Y_{it} = 0|\eta_{it}) = \exp(-\exp(\eta_{it}))$ and $P(Y_{it} = 1|\eta_{it}) = 1-\exp(-\exp(\eta_{it}))$. Assuming underlying Poisson variables $Y_{it}^\star, i = 1,...,n, t = 1,...,t_i$, so that $Y_{it} = I[Y_{it} > 0]$, it follows that

$$P(Y_{it} = 0|\eta_{it}) = P(Y_{it}^\star = 0|\eta_{it}) = \exp(-\exp(\eta_{it}))$$

and

$$P(Y_{it} = 1|\eta_{it}) = P(Y_{it}^\star > 0|\eta_{it}) = 1-\exp(-\exp(\eta_{it})).$$

The full conditional distribution of $Y_{it}^\star$ is a Poisson distribution with single parameter $\exp(\eta_{it})$ truncated from below at zero if $y_{it} = 1$ and degenerate at zero otherwise. Integrating $f(\boldsymbol{Y}^\star, \boldsymbol{\theta}|\mathscr{D})$ in $Y^\star$ yields $f(\boldsymbol{\theta}|\mathscr{D})$, so the introduction of the latent variable into a Gibbs sampler yields again a valid data augmentation scheme (Dunson and Herring 2004). An efficient method to obtain random deviates from the truncated Poisson distribution is given by Cumbus et al. (1996). While conditioning on Poisson distributed variables does not result in conditional conjugate distributions for most paramaters, conditioning on $\boldsymbol{Y}^\star$ nevertheless yields simplication as inference the Poisson likelihood is generally easier than dealing with the cloglog link. For IWLS proposals the expressions for the weights and working observations are very simple for Poisson data as the $\log(\cdot)$ is the natural link function for the Poisson distribution and due to the equivariance property of the Poisson distribution. The weight matrix is given by diag$(\mu_{11},...,\mu_{nt_n})$ and the working observations are

$$\dot{y}_{it} = \eta_{it} + y_{it}/\mu_{it} - 1, i = 1, ..., n, t = 1, ..., t_i,$$

where $\mu_{it} = \exp(\eta_{it}) = \text{var}(Y_{it}^{\star}|\eta_{it})$. Furthermore the Poisson likelihood is conditionally conjugate to a gamma prior, so that gamma frailties are an alternative to Gaussian random intercept models. Under the hazard

$$h(t|w_i, \boldsymbol{\theta}, \eta_{ij}) = 1 + \exp(-w_i \exp(\eta_{ij})), i = 1, ..., n, j = 1, ..., t_i,$$

where a priori $w_i \sim G(\kappa^{-1}, \kappa^{-1})$ with mean one and variance κ, the full conditional distribution of $w_i, i = 1, ..., n$ is

$$w_i \sim G(\kappa^{-1} + \sum_{j=1}^{t_i} y_{ij}, \kappa^{-1} + \sum_{j=1}^{t_i} \exp(\eta_{ij}))).$$

A hyperprior is usually assigned for κ, the full conditional distribution $f(\kappa|\cdot, \mathscr{D})$ is not conditionally conjugate. Drawing from the latent variables does not add much computational burden as draws only have to be obtained if $y_{it} = 1$, which for failure time data usually is the vast minority of data points.

5 Application I: Unemployment Durations

Discrete time models are applied on a data set of the NEPS panel study (Blossfeld et al. 2011). The data was obtained as retroperspective interviews. Analyzed are unemployment durations. As unemployment spells can be repeated, only the first unemployment spells are analyzed. Additionally, the transition from unemployment to employment is not exclusive; there are several types of failure. Applying the methods of this thesis is valid under the latent failure time approach: Here, spells that did not result into employment are taken as censored, hence it is assumed that there exists a latent employment failure time which is not observed (Crowder 2001, pp. 37–38). Some possible model improvements using methods not covered in this thesis are the inclusion of all spells via recurrent failure methods and the inclusion of all modes of failure. A complete case analysis is carried out. 773 individuals remain in the sample. The analysis was limited to spells whose beginning lies in the years 1995-2005. Spells lasting longer than 24 months are seen as censored. Estimation was carried out using a R-function appended as the thesis. Sampling of truncated normal deviates was done via the `rtruncnorm` function from the `truncnorm` package (Trautmann et al. 2012), which implements the sampler by Geweke (1991) and was found to be very stable. A first try, based on a inverse cdf approach was found to be unstable, sometimes producing infinite values.

The covariates used as fixed effects were:

- **sex** binary variable indicating sex=female
- **foreign** binary variable indicating for individuals with migration background
- **training** binary variable indicating that an individual was not born in Germany

Table 5.1: Model assessment

	LPML	DIC	p_D	deviance
grouped Cox	-2063.6	4093.5	33.4	4060.1
probit	-2085.7	4138.1	32.1	4105.9

- **registered** binary variable indicating registration of unemployment at begin of unemployment

These covariates were used for modeling of smooth effects via P-splines:

- **casmin** education years coded via casmin classification
- **time** process time
- **historical time** historical time, ranging from 2001 to 2011
- **age** age in years at beginning of unemployment spell

Furthermore, seasonality with perior length 12 was included, leading to the model

$$\begin{aligned} g(P(T = t|T \geq t, \eta)) = &\beta_0 + \beta_1 * sex + \beta_2 * foreigner + \beta_3 * training + \\ &\beta_4 * registered + f_0(time) + f(age) + f(casmin) + \\ &f(season) + f(historicaltime) \end{aligned}$$

A grouped Cox and a probit model were used. For the grouped Cox, sampling scheme 3 was used, additionally a completion Gibbs sampler with latent Poisson variables as described in section 4.2.3 in combination with sampling scheme 3 was tried. Truncated Poisson variables were sampled via the inverse cdf method using standard R-functions for the Poisson distribution. For the grouped Cox sampler there were very high correlations between the seasonal and the baseline hazard coefficients causing the sampler to get stuck (see figure 5.1), those parameters were drawn in one block. This was done by combining the design, penalty matrices and restriction matrices into blockmatrices. This resulted in lower acceptance rates (around 20%) which was found to be acceptable for a vector of size 171.

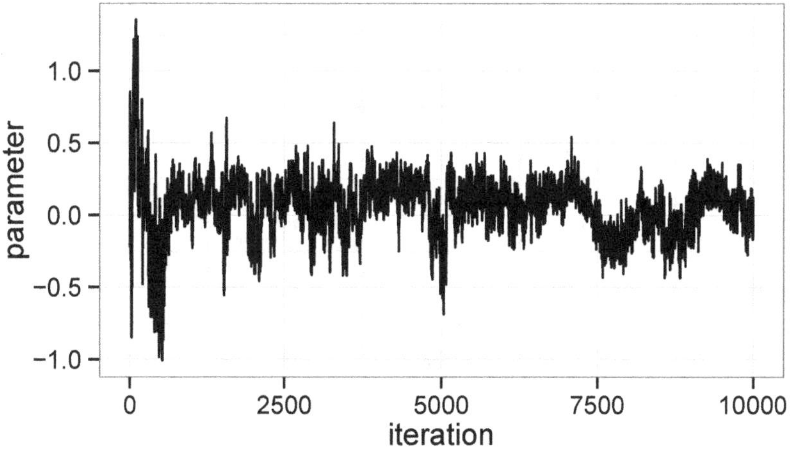

Figure 5.1: Convergence problems for unblocked parameter.

Sampling scheme 3 was found to behave somewhat erratically: There were long stretches where no draws were accepted, often after convergence seemed to have been reached see figure 5.6. Furthermore there were numerical problems due to the exponential functions involved in the complementary log-log link. It might be the case that sampling was not done long enough, for the completion Gibbs sampler this behaviour was not observed however, as such the results of this sampler are reported here. All in all, this sampler was much more stable. For other parameters, results of the samplers were very similar. Acceptance rates were around 50% for all parameters excluding baseline hazard coefficients.

For the probit model, no further adjustments were made and the standard sampler was used, using sampling scheme 4. The probit model achieves more indepedent draws than both sampler. A fair comparison would furthermore include execution times, as the sampler for the probit model is about 2 times faster although this depends on the implementation. For both models, 12000 iterations were used, the first 2000 were taken as burnin. Convergence could probably be accelerated by using better start values, here all parameters were set to zero at the

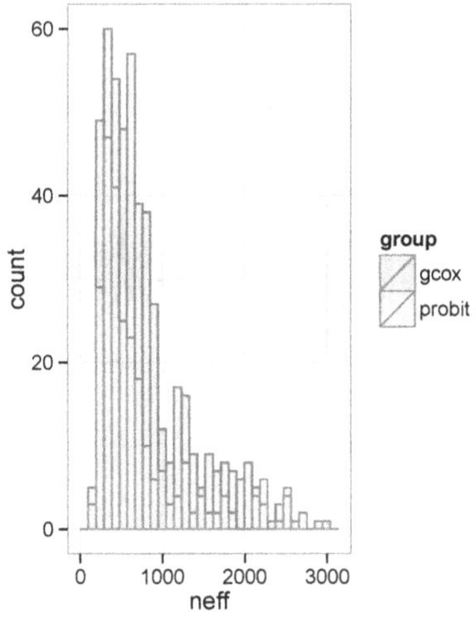

Figure 5.2: Histograms of numbers of effective parameter draws for both samplers.

beginning. It was noticed that convergence was heavily influenced by start values for the basis function coefficients and the corresponding variance parameter, which is part of the reason why one long chain was run instead of multiple independent chains. All in all, the influence of start-values seems to be a problem of IWLS proposals, this was also mentioned by Brezger and Lang (2006) who used a mode finding algorithm to find start values. Under all model diagnostics shown here, the grouped Cox model is preferable. This is not suprising as the complementary log-log link usually fits failure time data better to its asymmetry. The LPML statistic was computed using the harmonic mean estimator. Estimated nonlinear are given only for the grouped Cox model in figure 5.5, as the model fits better and results can be directly interpreted in terms of a latent failure time variable. Furthermore, results were very similar to the probit. All nonlinear effects were estimated using B-splines of degree 3 with 30 knots and a difference penalty of order 2.

The posterior quantiles of the baseline hazard are somewhat wide, probably owing the fact that time is decomposed into three effects, the estimates of which are not uncorrelated. We find slight negative duration dependence for the first

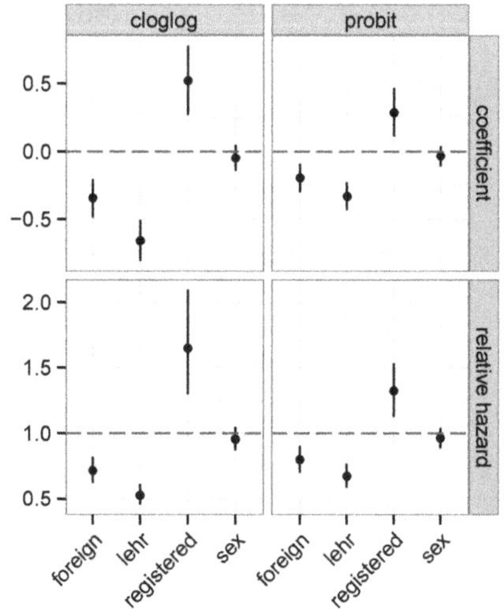

Figure 5.3: Relative hazards $P(T=t,z=1|T\geq t)/P(T=t,z=0|T\geq t)$ for both models. Estimates are averaged over time, keeping the other covariates at zero, including the constant at the posterior mean.

unemployment durations, so that the chance of leaving unemployment gets worse with the length of the unemployment spell. For seasonality, it is found that chance of finding employment is biggest at december, this seems implausible and might be related to data collection, this might well be a heaping effect. The effect of age shows that the B-spline fit could very well be replaced by a linear effect. For the effect of education it can be seen that the slope of the function starts out at approximately zero, followed by a positive effect around year 12. This however should not be overinterpreted due to the wide posterior quantiles. For the time trend, the effect peaks strongly around year 1999. The estimated seasonal effects are almost constant over time.

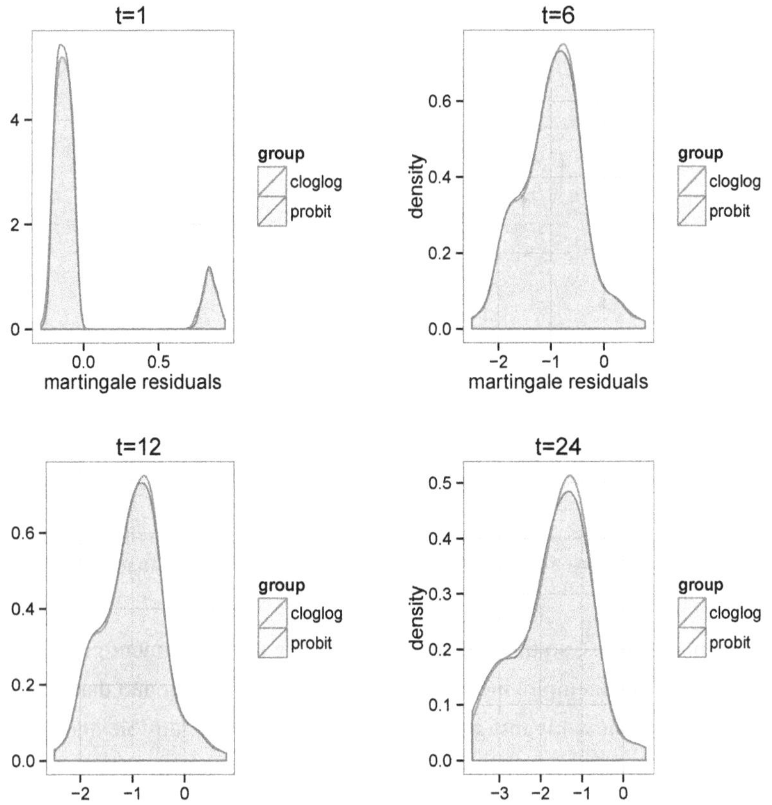

Figure 5.4: Density curves for martingale residuals at selected points in time. The grouped Cox model with complementary log-log link is can be seen to perform slightly better, the distribution of the residuals is more centered around zero for this model.

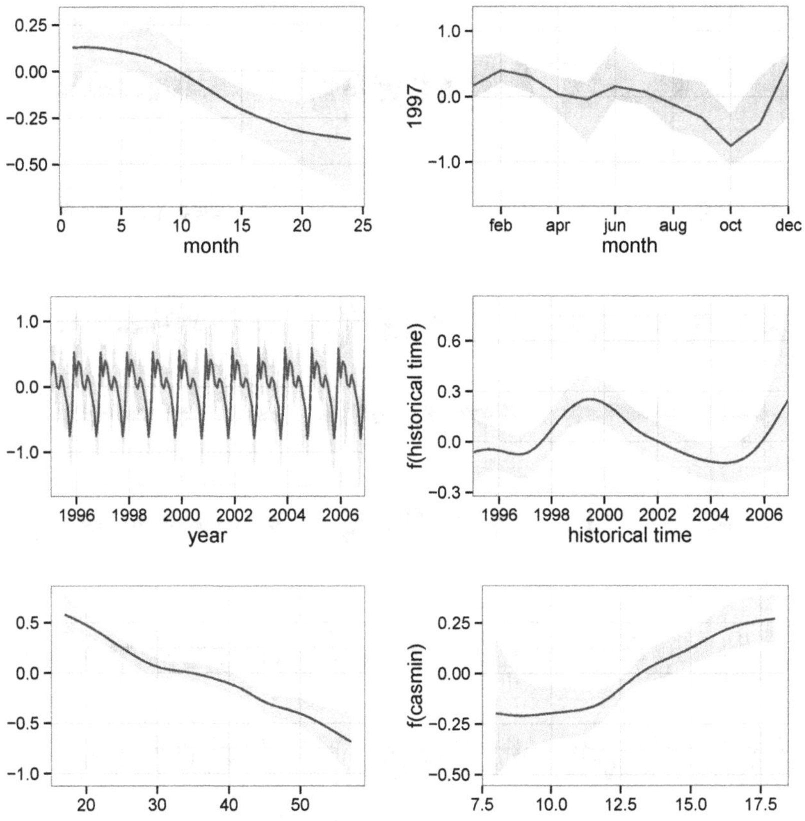

Figure 5.5: Estimated nonlinear effects with 5% and 95% posterior quantiles

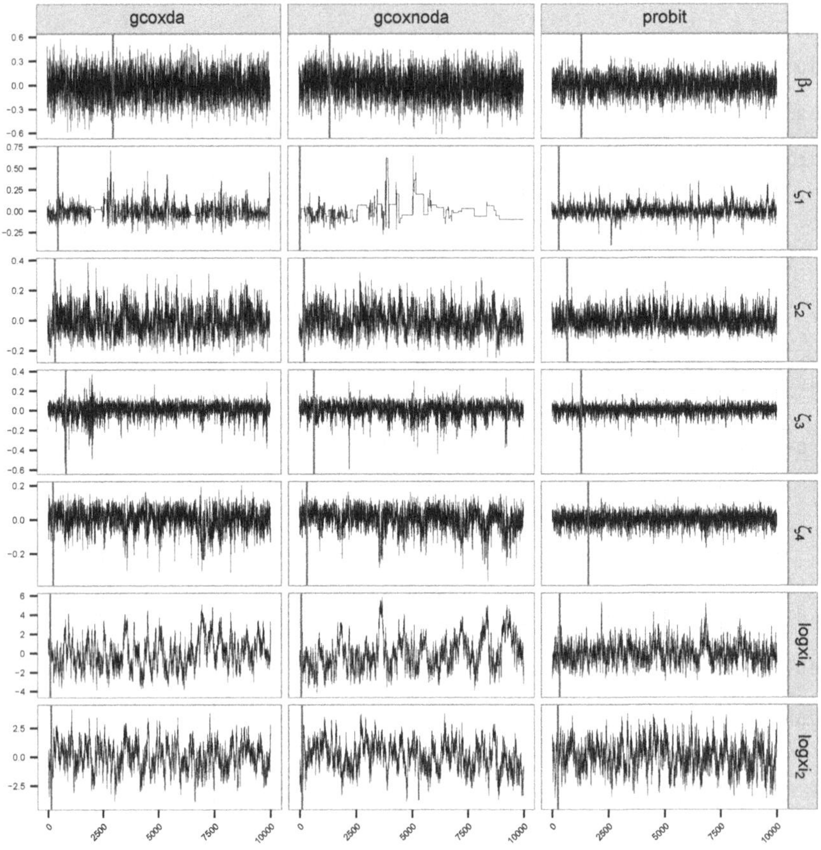

Figure 5.6: Trace plots for selected parameters. The results have been centered for visualization purposes. Left column, IWLS proposals with data augmentation, middle column IWLS proposals without, right column probit model.

6 Continuous Time Models

In this chapter, models for continuous time will be discussed. It is structured as follows: The lognormal model and some extensions based on it are discussed first, followed by relative risk models. For relative risk models, there is a unified approach for estimation based on IWLS proposals. The section on relative risk is split into a section on parametric relative risk models, where the baseline hazard is fully parameterized and nonparametric relative risk models, where the (log) baseline hazard is modeled via P-splines.

6.1 Lognormal and Extensions

The lognormal distribution is characterized by the following quantities:

$$\begin{aligned}\text{probability density function } f(t_i|\mu,\sigma) &= \frac{1}{t_i\sqrt{2\pi\sigma^2}}\exp(-\frac{1}{2\sigma^2}(\log t_i-\mu)^2)\\ \text{survivor function } g(t_i|\mu,\sigma) &= 1-\Phi(\frac{\log t_i-\mu}{\sigma}).\end{aligned}$$

Unlike many distributions which will be discussed in the following, the hazard of the lognormal distribution is nonmonotone and the support is given by $(0,\infty)$. The shape of the hazard is controlled by $\sigma > 0$, $\mu \in (-\infty,\infty)$ is a location parameter. As can be seen in figure 6.1 the lognormal hazard is zero at t=0, reaches a maximum and decreases in the following. This shape is often observed, e.g. for marriage dissolution by divorce (Lawless 2003, pp. 22–23). Covariates are usually introduced through $\mu_i = \eta_i$. As the expectation and median are given by $\exp(\mu_i + \sigma^2/2)$ and $\exp(\mu_i)$, parameter interpretation is straightforward in terms of those quantities, bot clearly not in terms of the hazard rate given by,

$$h(t_i|\mu,\sigma^2) = \left[\frac{1}{t_i\sqrt{2\pi\sigma^2}}\exp(-\frac{1}{2\sigma^2}(\log t_i-\mu_i)^2)\right] / \left[1-\Phi(\frac{\log t_i-\mu_i}{\sigma})\right].$$

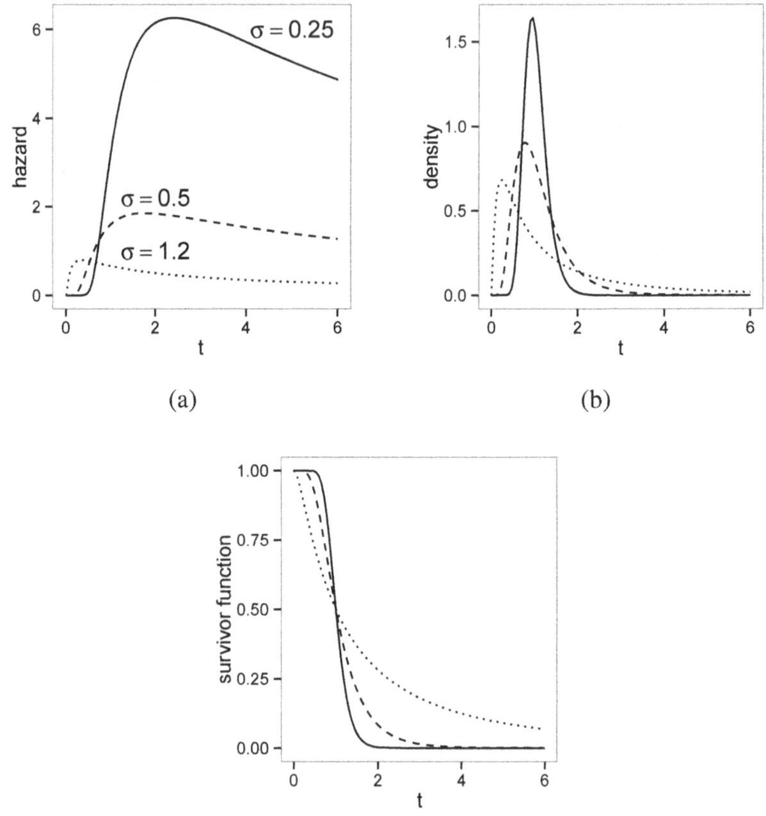

Figure 6.1: (a) hazard (b) density (c) survivor function of the lognormal distribution

Here the linear predictor for the lognormal model has the form

$$\boldsymbol{\eta} = \boldsymbol{Z\beta} + \boldsymbol{W\alpha} + \boldsymbol{B}_1(\boldsymbol{x}_1) + \ldots + \boldsymbol{B}_m(\boldsymbol{x}_m),$$

where no effect is allowed to depend on time and no time varying covariates are included. Working with the observed data likelihood under censoring usually involves Metropolis-Hastings steps, evaluation of the likelihood involves computation of Φ for censored failure times which must be done via numerical integration. A completion Gibbs sampler bypasses this problem, using the unknown failure times as latent variables. As $\log T = Y$ is distributed as $N(\mu, \sigma^2)$, a Gibbs sampler can be set on the log scale, which is easier (Sha et al. 2006). Sampling proceeds using sampling scheme 1 with an additional block for the latent failure times. This can be done for right and interval censoring, with data given by

$$D = \{([l_i, r_i), \mathbf{z}_i^\top)_{i=1}^n\},$$

where it is known that the failure occurs in the interval $[l_i, r_i)$. For all censored individuals, the latent data is drawn from $TN_{[\log l_i, \log r_i)}(\eta_i, \sigma^2)$. Given the complete data, the Gibbs sampler can proceed exactly as sampling scheme 1. A distribution from the family of scale-mixtures can be used, adding additional blocks for scale parameters. As robust alternative the t-distribution can be used for $\log T$. Furthermore using that $\log T$ is Gaussian, the available methodology for the normal distribution can be applied. Some relevant methods, which are beyond the scope of this thesis but should be mentioned are:

- Mixture of normal distributions for $\log T$ to achieve more flexibility.
- Multivariate modeling of failure time and longitudinal data using the multivariate normal distribution.

It should be noted that given complete data, many other distributions additionally used in failure time analysis belong to the exponential family. A completion Gibbs sampler combined with IWLS proposals for untractable conditionals might be applied, adding a block for additional parameters, using the response function $E[T_i|\eta_i] = \exp(\eta_i)$. This applies e.g. for the gamma and the inverse Gaussian distribution, which are sometimes used for failure time modeling.

6.2 Relative Risk Models

This section is concerned with regression models where the hazard can be written in the form

$$h(t_i|\eta_i,\Psi) = h_0(t_i|\Psi)\exp(\overline{\eta_i}) = \exp(\eta_i), \tag{6.1}$$

where $\overline{\eta_i}$ is the linear predictor without the effect of time, $\eta_i = \overline{\eta_i} + \log(h_0(t_i|\Psi))$ and $h_0(t_i|\Psi)$ is the baseline hazard, depending on Ψ. Time varying variables are possible but for now it is assumed that all covariates are constant over time. In this case, the likelihood for models with hazard rate 6.1 is

$$L = \prod_{i=1}^{n} L_i = \prod_{i=1}^{n} \{h_0(t_i)\exp(\overline{\eta_i})\}^{v_i} \exp(-\exp(\overline{\eta_i})H_0(t_i)),$$

where the conditioning in the likelihood on parameters is surpressed for notational simplicity and $H_0(t_i) = \int_0^{t_i} h_0(u)du$ is the cumulative baseline hazard. As shown by Aitkin and Clayton (1980), the likelihood can be written as:

$$\begin{aligned} L &= \prod_{i=1}^{n} L_i[\frac{H_0(t_i)}{H_0(t_i)}]^{v_i} \\ &= \prod_{i=1}^{n} [H(t_i)^{v_i} \exp(-H(t_i))] \left[\frac{h_0(t_i)}{H_0(t_i)}\right]^{v_i}, \end{aligned} \tag{6.2}$$

here

$$H(t_i) = \exp(\overline{\eta_i} + o_i) = \int_0^{t_i} \exp(\eta),$$

and $o_i = \log H_0(t_i|\Psi)$. Defining the censoring indicators as dependent variables, the likelihood 6.2 is proportional to a Poisson likelihood with log link and mean $H(t_i)$. For parametric relative risk models, $H_0(t_i)$ can usually be given in closed form. For left-truncated failure times, $H(t_i)$ is changed to

$$\log \int_{t_{ri}}^{t_i} h_0(u)\,du,$$

where t_{ri} is the truncation time and equals 0 for individuals with untruncated failure times. Hence time-varying covariates can be included by episode-splitting as described in section 2.3.2. Estimation can be done using sampling scheme 2 or 3 for Poisson responses, using linear predictor $\overline{\eta_i} + o_i$, for dependent variables $v_i, i = 1, ..., n$ with an additional block introduced for $\mathbf{\Psi}$ (Gamerman 1997). Weights are given by $\text{diag}(H(t_1), ..., H(t_n))$ and working observations

$$\dot{y}_i = \eta_i + v_i/H(t_i) - 1, i = 1, ..., n, \tag{6.3}$$

the proposal distribution, for example for $\boldsymbol{\zeta}_j$ with prior

$$f(\boldsymbol{\zeta}|\xi^2) \propto \exp(-\frac{1}{2\xi^2}\boldsymbol{\zeta}'\boldsymbol{K}\boldsymbol{\zeta})$$

is given as $N(\boldsymbol{m}_{\zeta_j}, \boldsymbol{\Sigma}_{\zeta_j)}$, with covariance matrix

$$\boldsymbol{\Sigma}_{\zeta_j} = [\boldsymbol{Z}^\top \boldsymbol{W}\boldsymbol{Z} + \boldsymbol{K}_j/\xi^2]^{-1},$$

and expectation

$$\boldsymbol{m}_{\zeta_j} = \boldsymbol{\Sigma}_{\zeta_j}(\boldsymbol{Z}^\top \boldsymbol{W}[\dot{\boldsymbol{y}} - \boldsymbol{\eta} + \boldsymbol{B}_j\boldsymbol{\zeta}_j]).$$

A tailored proposal for nonparametric relative risk models with linear predictor

$$\boldsymbol{\eta} = \boldsymbol{Z}\boldsymbol{\beta} + \boldsymbol{W}\boldsymbol{\alpha} + \boldsymbol{B}_1(x_1) + ... + \boldsymbol{B}_m(\boldsymbol{x}_m), \tag{6.4}$$

as for discrete time models was developed using steps analog to the development of IWLS proposals by Hennerfeind (2006). Here $\boldsymbol{x}_1 = \boldsymbol{t}$, $\boldsymbol{B}(t)$ describes the log-baseline and all basis functions are allowed to further depend on time, so that $h(\eta_i) = \exp(\eta_i)$. The proposal distribution was obtained by approximating the loglikelihood by a second order Taylor expansion around the current value $\boldsymbol{\zeta}_j^c$, giving the kernel of a multivariate normal distribution with covariance matrix and expectation given by

$$\boldsymbol{\Sigma}_j = (\boldsymbol{K}_j - \boldsymbol{H}(\boldsymbol{\zeta}_j^c))^{-1}, \boldsymbol{\mu}_j = \boldsymbol{\Sigma}_j[s(\boldsymbol{\zeta}_j^c) - \boldsymbol{H}(\boldsymbol{\zeta}_j^c)\boldsymbol{\zeta}_j^c],$$

where $\boldsymbol{H}$ is the Hesse matrix and $s(\boldsymbol{\zeta}_j^c)$ is the score vector. Plugging the expressions for the derivates, the proposal distribution can be represented in terms of working observations, which have the same form as 6.3; where

$$H(t_i) = \int_0^{t_i} \exp(\eta_i(u))\, du$$

for an untruncated and $\int_{t_{ri}}^{t_i} \exp(\eta_i(u))\, du$ for a truncated failure time. A general sampling scheme for relative risk models is given in the following:

Sampling scheme 6

1 Draw parameters by sampling scheme 2 using weights $H(t_1), ..., H(t_n))$ and working observations

$$\dot{y}_i = \eta_i + v_i / H(t_i) - 1, i = 1, ..., n$$

2 Draw $\boldsymbol{\Psi}$

Sampling scheme 3 might also be used for the first step although this does not seem to have been done in the literature. If there are no time varying effects and if the cumulative baseline hazard can be given in closed form, all necessary quantities can be calculated exactly. Otherwise, integrals of the form

$$\int_0^{t_i} \exp(\log h_0(t_i | \boldsymbol{\Psi}^{(s)}) + \sum \sum x_{ij} \zeta_i^{(s)} B_i(t_i))$$

have to be solved for the evaluation of the likelihood and to compute the weights. Hennerfeind (2006) uses numerical integration based on a trapezoid rule, which approximates an integral of the form $\int_l^u f(u)\, du$ by

$$\sum_{i=2}^{J} [k_i^\star - k_{i-1}^\star] \frac{f(k_i^\star) + f(k_{i-1}^\star)}{2},$$

with knots $k_1 = l < k_2 < ... < k_J = u$. For interval-censored data, data augmentation might principally be used if it is possible to obtain draws from the conditional distribution of the failure times, which conditional on the data are always truncated to $[l_i, r_i)$. For parameteric relative risk models $\boldsymbol{\Psi}$ is usually given by 1-2 positive parameters. A simple method to update these parameters via Metropolis-Hastings updates is to use a random walk on the log scale, which corresponds to a multiplicative random walk on the original scale (Dellaportas and Roberts 2003, p. 7). The acceptance probability is

$$\min(\frac{f(\alpha^p,\boldsymbol{\theta}|\mathscr{D})\alpha^p}{f(\alpha^c,\boldsymbol{\theta}|\mathscr{D})\alpha^c},1).$$

Another possibility, used for example by Konrath (2013) for the Weibull distribution, is the use of a gamma distribution centered around the current value as proposal distribution. More advanced algorithms like the slice sampler or adaptive reject sampling might also be used.

As for the grouped Cox model, frailties distributed a priori as $G(\kappa^{-1},\kappa^{-1})$ - with an appropriate hyperprior for κ - can always be used as the gamma distribution is conditional conjugate to the Poisson distribution (Henschel et al. 2009). For the hazard

$$h_i(t_j) = h_0(t_j)\exp(\eta_{ij})w_i, i = 1,...,I, j = 1,...,n_i,$$

the conditional distribution for frailties $w_i, i = 1,...,J$ is

$$w_i \sim G(\kappa^{-1} + \sum_{j=1}^{n_i} v_{ij}, \kappa^{-1} + \sum_{j=1}^{n_i} \exp(o_i + \eta_{ij})),$$

where o_i is the integral 6.2 for the full predictor 6.4. In the following, some important distributions from the relative risk family are discussed. Estimation for these can always proceed using sampling scheme 6, with linear predictor 6.3 where $\boldsymbol{B}(\boldsymbol{t})$ is replaced by a closed form expression for $\log(h_0(\boldsymbol{t}))$. The support of all discussed distributions is given by $[0,\infty)$.

6.2.1 Exponential Distribution

Under the exponential distribution the hazard rate is given by the single parameter $h(t_i|\Upsilon) = \Upsilon$. The distribution is characterized by the following quantities:

$$\begin{aligned}
\text{probability density function } f(t_i|\Upsilon) =& \Upsilon \exp(-t_i\Upsilon)\\
\text{survivor function } G(t_i|\Upsilon) =& \exp(-t_i\Upsilon)\\
\text{cumulative hazard rate } H(t_i|\Upsilon) =& t_i\Upsilon\\
\text{hazard rate } h(t_i|\Upsilon) =& \Upsilon\\
\text{expectation } E(T_i|\Upsilon) =& \frac{1}{\Upsilon}.
\end{aligned}$$

Due to the fact that the hazard rate is constant over time, it holds that the distribution has a property called lack of memory:

$$G(T > t + x|T > x) = G(t).$$

The exponential distribution is a special case of the Weibull distribution if the corresponding shape parameter equals 1, see figure 6.2. Writing $\Upsilon = \exp(\beta_0)$, the hazard is $\exp(\eta)$, so that $h_0(t_i) = 1$ and o_i is given by $\log \int_0^t 1\,du = \log t_i, i = 1, ..., n$ for time-constant effects, which is free of additional paramaters, hence for a Gibbs sampler $o_i, .i = 1, ..., n$ can be computed at iteration 1 and stay unchanged. The ratio $h_0(t_i)/H_0(t_i) = 1/t_i$ in the likelihood 6.2 is a multiplicative constant that is free of parameters and can be ignored.

Assuming a time-constant hazard is often a stark oversimplification, the distribution is nevertheless of practical importance: Predictions based on the exponential have been shown to be more robust against misspecification, compared to distributions with more complicated hazard rates. The distribution is often used in this context, especially in the absence of covariates or when the inclusion of covariates is problematic (Thall et al. 2005). Under right censoring for a homogenous population, the distribution is conjugate to the gamma distribution. Under a $G(\alpha_0, \psi_0)$ prior for Υ, the posterior distribution of Υ is $G(\alpha_0 + d, \psi_0 + \sum_i^n t_i)$. Furthermore the posterior predictive distribution is available in closed form and given by an inverse beta distribution (Ibrahim et al. 2001b, pp. 31–32).

The distribution can be used as building block to more complex models. The exponential model can be generalized to the piecewise exponential model discussed in 6.3.1, where the time axis is partitioned into intervals and the hazard is assumed to be constant in every interval. Another generalization is the hyperexponential distribution, which is a mixture of exponential distribution, and does not have a relative risk hazard.

6.2.2 Weibull Distribution

The Weibull distribution is probably the most widely used distribution for failure time analysis. Use of the distribution can be motivated by the fact that the minimum of i.i.d. random variables can be shown to be approximately Weibull distributed. The random variables can be viewed as failure times associated with different causes of failure competing with each other, so that their minimum is the observed failure time (Wienke 2010, p. 31). In a relative risk context, the distribution is characterized by the following quantities:

$$\begin{aligned}
\text{probability density function } f(t_i|\alpha,\gamma) &= \alpha\gamma t_i^{\alpha-1}\exp(-\gamma t_i^{\alpha}) \\
\text{survivor function } G(t_i|\alpha,\gamma) &= \exp(-\gamma t_i^{\alpha}) \\
\text{cumulative hazard rate } H(t_i|\alpha,\gamma) &= \gamma t_i^{\alpha} \\
\text{hazard rate } h(t_i|\alpha,\gamma) &= \gamma\alpha t_i^{(\alpha-1)} \\
\text{expectation } E[T_i|\alpha,\gamma] &= \alpha^{-1/\gamma}\Gamma(1+\frac{1}{\gamma}),
\end{aligned}$$

where $\Gamma(s)=\int_0^\infty x^{s-1}\exp(-x)dx$ is the gamma function. The linear predictor is usually introduced through $\log(\gamma_i)=\eta_i$ so that $h_0(t_i)=\alpha t_i^{\alpha-1}$. The Weibull distribution is the only distribution with relative risk hazard that is also a member of the log-location-scale family. The variable $\log T_i = Y_i$ can be written as

$$Y_i = \eta_i^\star + \sigma W_i,$$

where $\sigma = 1/\alpha$ and $\eta_i^\star = -\sigma\eta_i$, and W_i follows the standard extrem value distri-

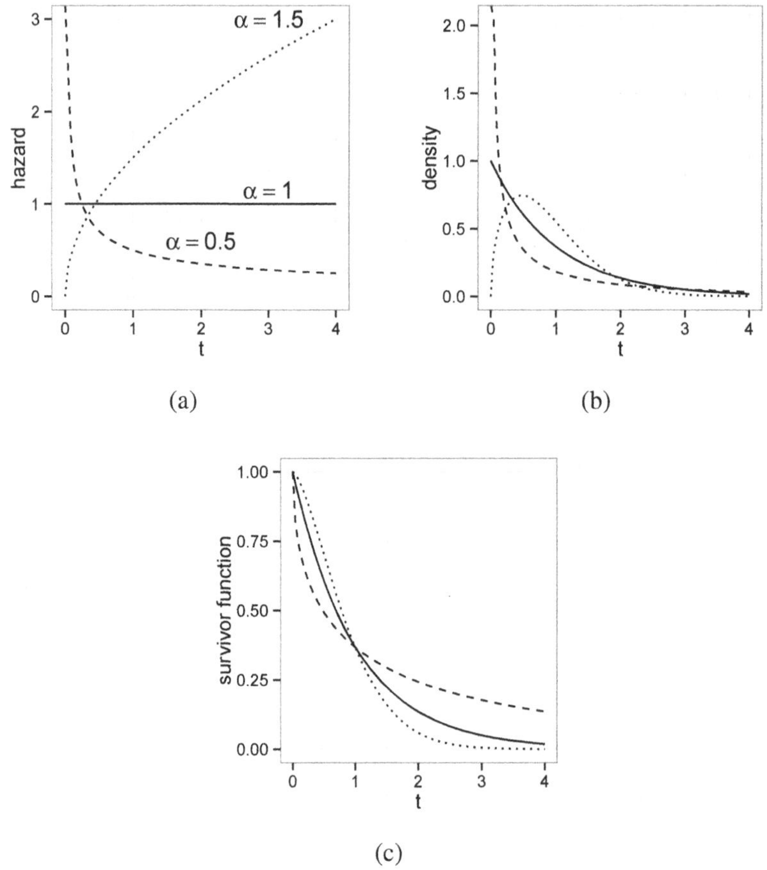

Figure 6.2: (a) hazard (b) density (c) survivor function of the Weibull distribution

bution from the location-scale distribution with pdf $f_W(y) = \exp(y - \exp(y))$.

As such parameter interpretation is possible in terms of the hazard and the failure time. The distribution is relatively flexible. The parameter α controls the shape of the hazard rate: For $\alpha > 1$ the hazard is monotonically increasing, for $0 < \alpha < 1$ it is monotonically decreasing (see figure 6.2), for $\alpha = 1$ a time-constant hazard is obtained giving the exponential distribution as special case. A gamma prior is often used for α. To capture hazards of other shapes, many extensions of the Weibull distribution have been proposed, these are discussed by Murthy et al. (2004).

6.2.3 Other Baseline Hazards

Other distributions with relative risk hazards but somewhat limited usability are the Gompertz and the Pareto distribution. The Gompertz baseline hazard is $\exp(\rho t)$, $\rho \in (-\infty, \infty)$. As such the distribution is appropriate exclusively for applications with exponentially growing hazard - a major application is modeling of human adult mortality. The Pareto distribution has baseline hazard $(w+t)^{-1}$ and survivor function $((1+t/w)^{-1})^{\exp(\eta_i)}$, w>0. This hazard shape is not very interesting, the defining property of the distribution are its wide tails which might make the distribution attractive for robust modeling of outliers. Both the Gompertz and the Pareto distribution can be defective for certain parameter values (Wienke 2010, pp. 33–37). A relative risk hazard with a nonmonotone baseline hazard which is always nondefective is given by the sickle model by Diekmann and Mitter (1983). The hazard is given by $h(t|a,b) = a\exp(\log t - \frac{t}{b})$, a,b>0. The shape of the hazard is similar to the lognormal distribution. The survival fraction is $\exp(-ab^2)$. Covariates can be introduced via $a_i = \exp(\eta_i)$.

A hazard of the form 6.1 for a nondefective random variable can always be produced by using an appropriate function for $h_0(t_i|\Psi)$, so the approach is actually fairly flexible. The baseline hazard might be generated by theoretical considerations, for example Flinn and Heckman (1982) use

$$h_0(t_i|\Psi) = \exp(\gamma_0 + \gamma_1 \frac{t_i^{\lambda_1} - 1}{\lambda_1} + \gamma_2 \frac{t_i^{\lambda_2} - 1}{\lambda_2}),$$

based on the Box-Cox-transformation, derived from considerations regarding duration dependence. A convenient choice is to use the hazard of an arbitrary distribution for h_0 (Cox and Oakes 1984, p. 73). Under this approach the resulting density in general does not correspond to a known distribution. Draws from the predictive distributions can still be obtained by the method described in 3.3 in the context of the L-measure, using the hazard rate.

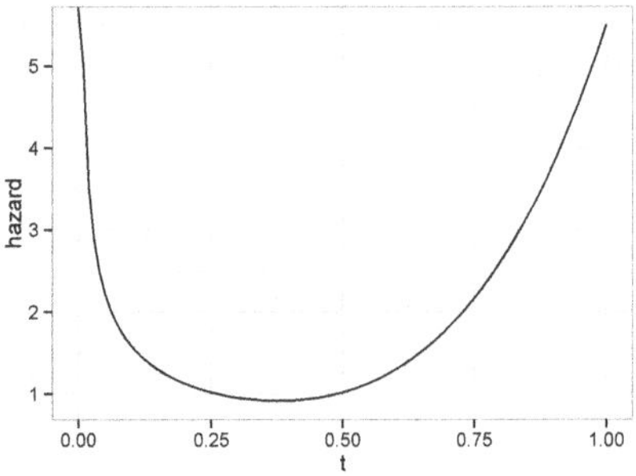

Figure 6.3: Example of a bathtub shaped hazard

6.3 Nonparametric Relative Risk Models

The flexibility of parametric models is for many applications insufficient. For example many hazard shapes observed in practice can be described as bathtub-shaped (Bebbington et al. 2006): Here the hazard consists of a decreasing part, followed by approximately constant hazard, followed by an increasing hazard, see figure 6.3. None of the aforementioned distributions can give such a hazard without adjustments. While a distribution corresponding to a specific shape of hazard usually can be found, it is often preferable to estimate the hazard from the data by flexible methods, especially under the absence of information about the shape of the hazard. In the following such nonparametric models are discussed.

6.3.1 Piecewise Exponential Hazard

The piecewise constant model is a simple but useful model, for which estimation is relatively easy and interval-censoring can be accounted for. The time axis is partioned into m intervals $[s_0 = 0, s_1), [s_1, s_2), ..., [s_{m-1}, s_m = \infty)$. The baseline hazard in every interval is approximated by a constant, the hazard of an exponential distribution:

$$h_0(t) = \begin{cases} \lambda_1 & \text{if } t \in [s_0, s_1) \\ \lambda_2 & \text{if } t \in [s_1, s_2) \\ \vdots & \\ \lambda_m & \text{if } t \in [s_{m-1}, s_m). \end{cases}$$

Lawless (2003, p. 385) shows that if the number of knots tends to infinity, the conditional likelihood of all regression coefficients is given by

$$\prod_{i=1}^{d} \frac{\exp(\eta_i)}{\sum_{j \in \mathscr{R}(i)} \exp(\eta_i)},$$

the partial likelihood, see chapter 2.4. Hence for a large number of knots, estimates from piecewise constant model should approximately agree with estimates based on partial likelihood.

The baseline hazard depends on $\boldsymbol{\Psi} = (\lambda_1, ..., \lambda_m)^\top$. The likelihood contributions under right censoring are

$$h_i^{v_i} \exp(-\sum_{j=1}^{m} d_j h_{ij}),$$

where $h_i = h_0(t_i)\exp(\eta(t_i))$, $\sum_{j=1}^{m} d_j h_{ij}$ is the cumulative hazard rate and $d_{ij} = \min(t_i, s_b) - s_{b-1}$ is the time individual i spent in interval j. The likelihood is

$$L = \prod_{i=1}^{n} \prod_{j=1}^{m} (h_i)^{v_{ij}} \exp(-d_{ij} h_{ij}). \tag{6.5}$$

As shown by Laird and Olivier (1981) and Holford (1980), 6.5 is proportional to a Poisson likelihood with dependent variables given by $v_{ij} = I[t_i \in [s_{j-1}, s_j)]$ and offsets $\log d_{ij}, i = 1, ..., n, j = 1, ..., m$. Hence, in analogy to the models of section 6.2, GLM methodology as described in 4.1 can be applied. The data set must be expanded similar as for discrete time models, as can be seen in table 6.1. On the left is a data set before expansion, on the right after expansion.

Time varying covariates can be included by varying covariate values between the intervals. The parameters $\log \lambda_1, \log \lambda_2, ..., \log \lambda_m$ and piecewise constant varying time-dependent effects can be estimated using P-splines of order 0. The knot

Table 6.1: Data set expansion for piecewise constant model, given knots 0, 2, 5, 8

id	t	v	z1	id	interval	v	z1	offset
1	4	0	3	1	1	0	3	1.1
2	5.3	1	5	1	2	0	3	.7
				2	1	0	5	1.1
				2	2	0	5	1.1
				2	3	1	5	-1.2

placement strategy given in section 3.4.1 can be used to determine the intervals. Of course the model can also be estimated without the data expansion. An alternative to the normal prior for $\log\lambda_1,\ldots,\log\lambda_m$ is the use of a gamma prior for $\lambda_1,\ldots,\lambda_m$. Similar to the random walk prior for P-splines, correlation can be induced to penalized abrupt jumps. For example, Aslanidou et al. (1998) use

$$\lambda_k|\lambda_{k-1},\lambda_{k-2},\ldots,\lambda_1 \sim G(\kappa_k,\frac{\kappa_k}{\lambda_{k-1}}),$$

the variance parameter κ_k controls the penalization.

Strictly speaking, the piecewise constant model is a fully parametric model, as a piecewise exponential distribution generalizing the exponential distribution can be defined. Under interval-censoring, unknown failure times can be drawn from this distribution for the construction of a completion Gibbs sampler. This approach has been used by Henschel et al. (2009) in connection with IWLS proposals. A draw from $f(t_i|\mathscr{D},\boldsymbol{\theta})$ can be obtained by a two-step procedure. Suppose it is known that t_i lies between $a_0 = L_i < a_1 < \ldots < a_p = R_i$, where $a_2,\ldots,a_{p-1}$ are knots. A draw can be obtained as follows (Wang et al. 2012b):

Sampling from the truncated exponential distribution

1 Determine the interval by drawing $(i_1,\ldots,i_{p-1})$ from a multinomial distribution with parameter $\boldsymbol{\alpha} = (\alpha_1,\ldots,\alpha_{p-1})^\top$ and size 1, where $\alpha_k \propto G(a_{k-1}) - G(a_k)$, if $i_k = 1$, the failure time is drawn from $[a_{k-1},a_k)$

2 Conditional on i_k, draw the failure time from an exponential distribution with rate $\lambda_i \exp(\eta_{ik})$, truncated to the interval $[a_{k-1},a_k)$

For step 2, draws from a truncated piecewise exponential distribution can be easily obtained by the inverse cdf method as the inverse of a cdf of the truncated exponential distribution can be found closed form.

6.3.2 Nonparametric Relative Risk Models

The underlying baseline hazard is rarely a step function, so approximating it by a smooth function is often more appropriate. A natural extension of the piecewise exponential model is the use of splines of higher order. Estimation proceeds using sampling scheme 6, here $\boldsymbol{\Psi}$ is given by a block of spline-coefficients corresponding to the matrix of basis functions $B(t)$. Proof of propriety of the posterior distribution under fairly general conditions is given by Hennerfeind et al. (2006). Noted by Hennerfeind (2006) are some computational complications and adjustments. For splines of order > 1, numerical integration is always necessary. For P-splines of order 1, corresponding to a piecewise Gompertz model, an analytical solution is possible but very cumbersome to compute so that numerical integration is preferable. As a simpler alternative to IWLS proposals, conditional prior proposals (Knorr-Held 1999) can be used for regression coefficients corresponding to basis functions depending on time. Giving the conditional mean of the prior in terms of standart formulae for the multivariate normal distribution is not possible, as the prior is not proper. The conditional moments can instead be given in terms of the penalty matrix (Fahrmeir and Lang 2000):

Supressing most indices for simplicity, suppose the subblock

$$\boldsymbol{\zeta}[r:s] = (\zeta_r, \zeta_{r+1}, ..., \zeta_s)^\top, r \leq s$$

from $\boldsymbol{\zeta} = (\zeta_1, ..., \zeta_{r-1}, \zeta_r ... \zeta_s, \zeta_{s+1}, ..., \zeta_m)^\top$ is updated. Let $\boldsymbol{K}[r:s, r:s]$ denote the submatrix of the penalty matrix corresponding to $\boldsymbol{\zeta}[r:s]$, so that $\boldsymbol{K}[r:s, 1:r-1]$ and $\boldsymbol{K}[r:s, s+1:m]$ are the matrices to the left and to the right. The conditional expectation of $\boldsymbol{\zeta}[r:s]$ given all remaining $\boldsymbol{\zeta}$ is:

$$E[\boldsymbol{\zeta}[r:s]|\cdot] = \begin{cases} -\xi^2\boldsymbol{K}[r:s,r:s]^{-1}\boldsymbol{K}[r:s,(s+1):m]\boldsymbol{\zeta}[s+1:m] & \text{if r} = 1 \\ -\xi^2\boldsymbol{K}[r:s,r:s]^{-1}\boldsymbol{K}[r:s,1:(r-1)]\boldsymbol{\zeta}[1:(r-1)] & \text{if s=m} \\ -\xi^2\boldsymbol{K}[r:s,r:s]^{-1}\{\boldsymbol{K}[r:s,(s+1):m]\boldsymbol{\zeta}[s+1:m]+ & \\ \qquad \boldsymbol{K}[r:s,1:(r-1)]\boldsymbol{\zeta}[1:(r-1)]\} & \text{else.} \end{cases}$$

The conditional variance is $\xi^2\boldsymbol{K}[r:s,r:s]^{-1}$. Here, the acceptance probability for Metropolis-Hastings update steps simplifies to

$$\alpha(\boldsymbol{\beta}^p,\boldsymbol{\beta}^c) = \min(\frac{L(\boldsymbol{\beta}_p^{\beta})}{L(\boldsymbol{\beta}_c^{\beta})},1),$$

the ratio of likelihoods. This simplifies computation but mixing is worse compared to IWLS proposals. Autocorrelation can be decreased by letting the blocksize vary randomly between iterations. An alternative approach might be to use sampling scheme 3 where the moments of the proposal distribution only have to be computed once.

A simpler, approximate approach is used by Lambert and Eilers (2005). Here the time axis $[0,\tau]$, where τ is the maximal observed failure time, is partitioned into intervals - here called bins - $I_j, j = 1,...,J$ with midpoints $\Delta_1,...,\Delta_J$. In every interval the number of failures follows a Binomial distribution with parameters e_j given by the number of failures in bin j and p_j given by the probability of failure in bin j. The authors use a large number of intervals and approximate the binomial distribution by a Poisson distribution with parameter $\mu_j = r_j p_j$, where r_j are the number of individuals at risk during interval j and use P-splines to smooth $p_1,...,p_J$. Based on a similar approach, Yavuz and Lambert (2011) estimate the parameters of the basic proportional hazard model under interval censoring. Under the PH model we have,

$$G(t_i|\boldsymbol{z},\boldsymbol{\beta}) = \exp(-\int_0^{t_i} h(u|\boldsymbol{z},\boldsymbol{\beta})) = \exp(-H_0(t_i)\exp(\eta_i)) = G_0(t_i)^{\exp(\eta_i)},$$

and

$$G_0(t_i) = 1 - \int_0^{t_i} f_0(u)\,du. \tag{6.6}$$

The binning approach is used to model f_0. Here

$$p_j = P(L_i < T_i < R_i|\mathbf{z} = 0) = \int_{I_j} f_0(u)\, du$$

is approximated by $f_0(u_j)\Delta_j$, where Δ_j is the midpoint of interval I_j. Then, the likelihood contribution of an individual with standard conditions $\mathbf{z} = 0$ can be written as

$$l_i = \sum_{i=J} p_j v_{ij} + d_j(1-\alpha), \tag{6.7}$$

where $v_{ij} = I[t_i \in I_j]$, $d_j = I[R_i > \tau]$ and $\alpha = P(T_i > \tau|\mathbf{z} = 0)$. Then, $P(t_i \in I_j|\mathbf{z} = 0)$ is estimated via P-splines coefficients $\zeta_1, ..., \zeta_k$ by

$$\hat{p}_j = \hat{\alpha}\frac{\exp(\gamma_j)}{\exp(\gamma_1) + ... + \exp(\gamma_J)},$$

where $\gamma_j = \sum_{p=1}^{k} \hat{\zeta}_p B_p(u_j)$. It follows that $f_0(t) \approx p_j/\Delta_j$, so that the likelihood contribution

$$l_i = G(l_i|\mathbf{z},\boldsymbol{\beta}) - G(r_i|\mathbf{z},\boldsymbol{\beta}) = G_0(l_i)^{\exp(\eta_i)} - G_0(r_i)^{\exp(\eta_i)}$$

is derived by plugging $p_j/\Delta_j = f_0$ into 6.6. Yavuz and Lambert (2011) use Gaussian random walk proposals on a reparametrized posterior distribution to explore the posterior. An exact, fully Bayesian application of the relative risk model under interval censoring does not seem to have been developed yet.

7 Application II: Crime Recidivism

In the second application, a data set on crime recidivism is used. The data set has been previously analyzed and obtained by Schmidt and Witte (1988). The data was obtained from files on inmates of a North Carolina prison who were released between July 1979 until June 1980. It can be freely downloaded from the webpage `https://www.icpsr.umich.edu/icpsrweb/ICPSR/studies/8987?q=ICPSR` as of 06/27/2014. The data set was assembled in 1984, the observation windows equals 81 month. The original sample is of size 9327, after deleting missing values 4628 cases remain. Failure time is defined as time until return to prison. Due to rounding, the failure times are interval-censored. Failure times are rounded to the nearest month, so that return to prison after 15 days would be coded 1, return after 16 days until the 15th of the following month would be coded 2. The month of release in addition to the month of return to prison are available, so the exact interval in which return to prison occured can be reconstructed. The covariates used for fixed effects in the model are

- **white** binary variable indicating if an individual is white[1] (referance category)
- **drugs** binary variable indicating if an individual's prison records indicates a serious problem with hard drugs or alcohol (before entering prison)
- **married** binary variable indicating if an individual was married at the time of prison entry
- **felony** binary variable indicating if an individual's crime was a felony (reference category: crime against a person)

[1] Using the coding of Schmidt and Witte (1988), all non-blacks are coded as whites.

Table 7.1: Model assessment

	LPML	DIC	p_D	deviance
piecewise constant	-8691.622	17357.72	25.35715	17332.36
lognormal	-9109.098	18118	54.52985	18064.26

- **workprogram** binary variable indicating if an individual's took part in a program aiding job search
- **supervised** binary variable indicating if an individual was supervised after release (for example for parole)
- **property** binary variable indicating if an individuals crime was against a property (reference category: crime against a person)
- **other** binary variable indicating crimes neither against a person nore against a property (reference category: crime against a person)

Furthermore, following covariates are modeled as smooth functions via P-splines:

- **rule violations** number of prison rule violations per month during the prison stay
- **age** age, in years at time of release
- **school years** number of formal schooling years
- **time served** time served (in months) for prison sentence

For the nonlinear effects, a difference penalty of order 2 with 30 knots were used for all function estimates. 8000 iterations were run, the first 1000 were taken as burnin.

A lognormal and a piecewise constant model were fitted. The lognormal model was chosen as a nonmonotone hazard seems more plausible than a monotone for this process. The usual inverse gamma prior was used for σ^2 with hyperparameter set to 0.001. For the piecewise constant model, a completion gibbs sampler

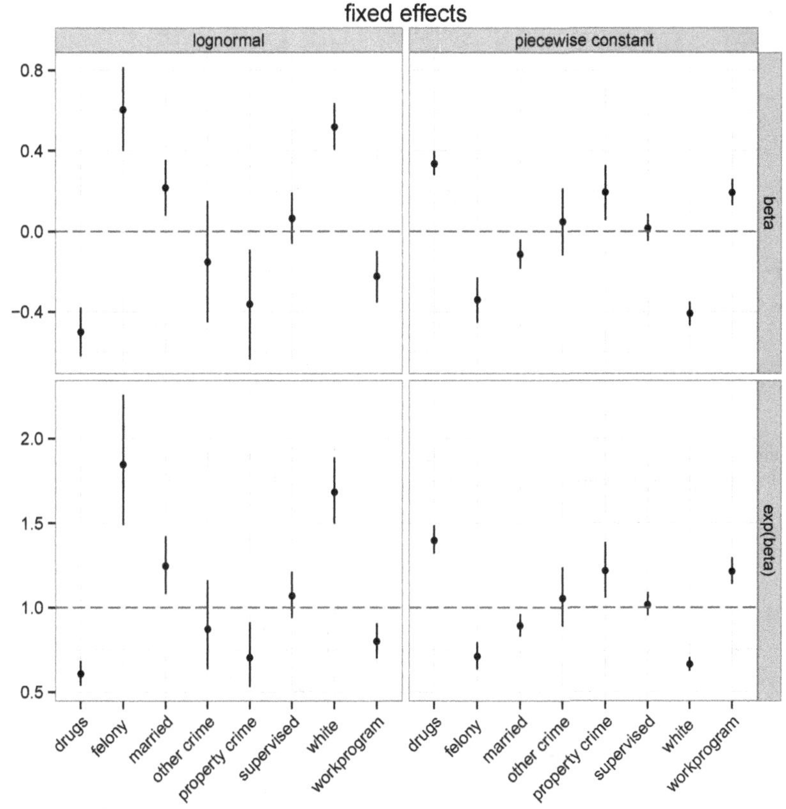

Figure 7.1: Estimated fixed effects for both models with 5% and 95% quantiles. The effects for the lognormal model are on the failure time, the effects of the piecewise constant hazard on the hazard rate.

based on a data-expansion with an additional block for failure times as described in section 6.3.1 was used. Sampling of failure times slows down the sampler considerably, however. Finding the interval in which the failure time lies was the most elaborate part, after this is achieved the sampling of the truncated exponential distribution can be quickly done by the inverse cdf method. The sampling scheme for the lognormal model is based on sampling scheme 1, with additional block for the logfailure times. As for the probit model, sampling of the latent failure time adds

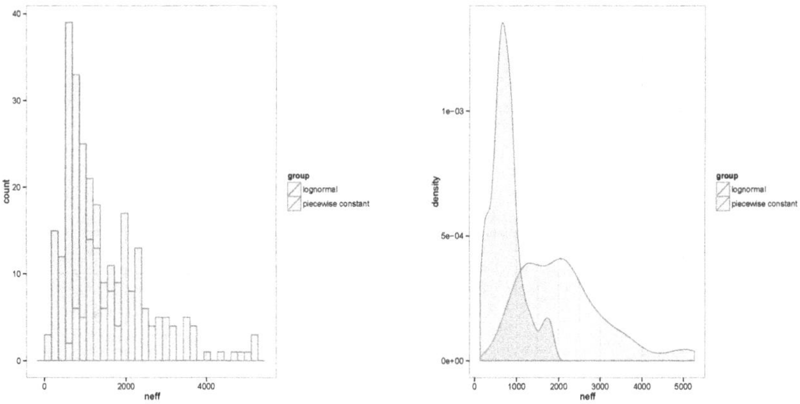

Figure 7.2: Histograms and kernel density estimates for the effective number of parameters, obtained via the `coda` package (Plummer et al. 2006).

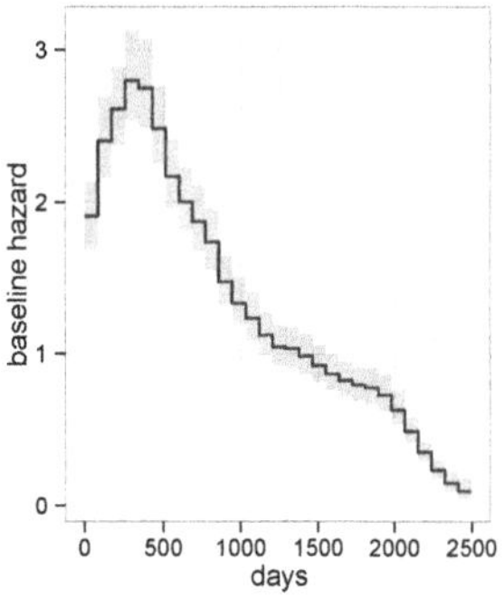

Figure 7.3: Baseline hazard for the piecewise constant model with 5% and 95% quantiles.

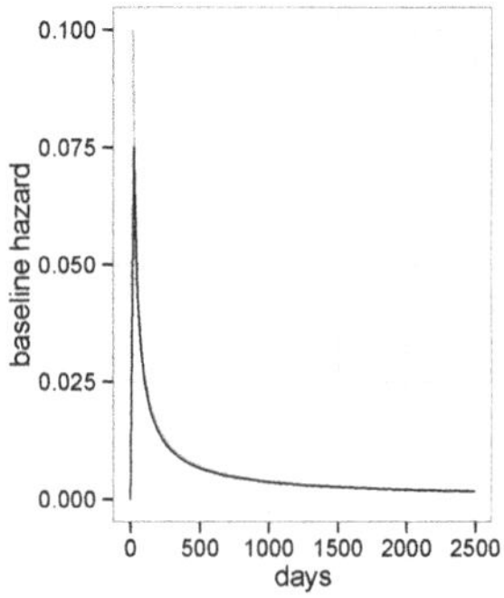

Figure 7.4: Baseline hazard for the lognormal model with 5% and 95% posterior quantiles. Note that the posterior quantiles for the lognormal model are very narrow and barely visible.

hardly and computational burden is done via the function `rtruncnorm`. Both were again implemented in R.

Diffuse priors were assigned to all fixed effects. The baseline hazard was estimated using a sum-to-zero constraint which seemed more natural here.

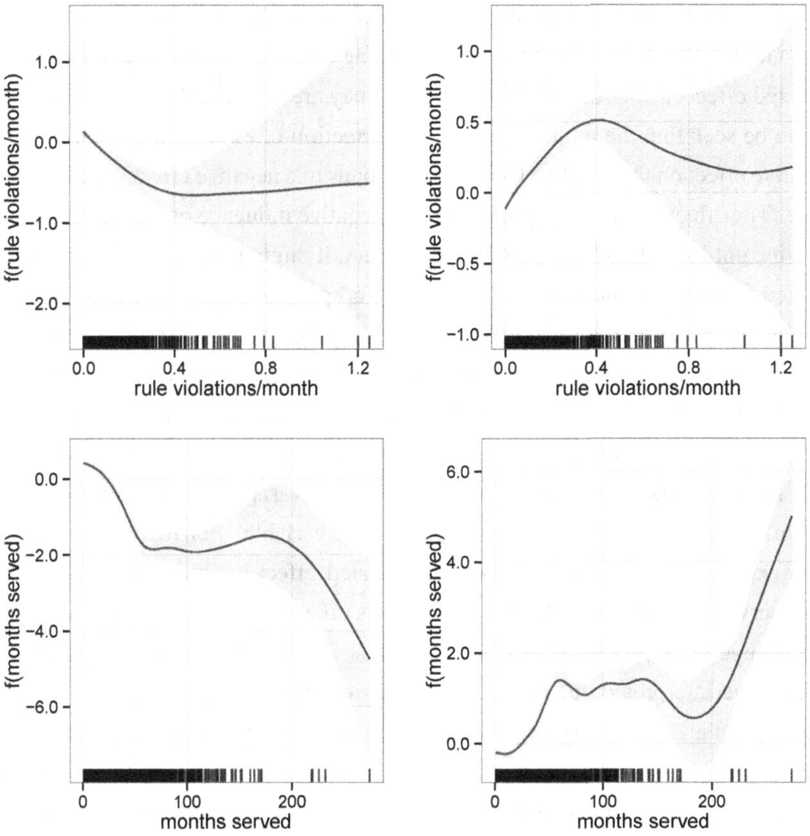

Figure 7.5: Estimated effects for both models with 5% and 95% posterior quantiles. The stripes represent unique observations. Left column: lognormal, right column: piecewise constant.

Mixing wise, the sampling scheme for the piecewise constant model did not perform very well, some selected sampling paths showing this can be seen in 7.7. This is probably due to the fact that the baseline coefficients are very strongly influenced by the latent failure times and vice versa. Estimated baseline hazard can be seen in 7.3 and 7.4. The LPMPL and the DIC favor strongly the more flexible piecewise constant model.

Surprisingly, the model complexity term of the DIC is lower for the piecewise constant model which is due to lower smoothing variances of this model. Estimates of fixed effects are visualized in figure 7.1. They are not directly comparable, still it can be seen that the models agree on the direction of effects, in the sense that a positive effect on the baseline hazard corresponds to a negative effect for the failure time. The effects seem mostly sensible; the negative influence of the workprogram on time until return to prison does seem suspect, it might be an artifact or might be related to the assignment procedure for the workprogram.

The estimated nonlinear effects can be seen in figure 7.6 and 7.5. The same inverse relation between hazard of piecewise constant and failure time of lognormal variable holds here. As can be seen some of these estimated effects are driven by individuals with very large covariate values, leading to very large posterior intervals for sparse data regions as it is the case for the variable rule violations, where the effects for sparse data regions become very variable. For regions with more data (<0.5 rule violations/month), the estimated effect is almost linear. For the time served, it can be seen that the effect levels off around circa 5 years of jail time, the change in slope for the piecewise constant model around 150 months should not be overinterpreted due to the large posterior interval. The nonlinear effect of age is estimated with very little variance and seems very sensible: Imprisonment during younger years should be much more disruptive compared to later years. In conclusion it can be said that the models agree with the general direction of effects but that the piecewise constant model fits better.

An alternative modeling approach should be mentioned. An interesting question might be if individuals return to prison at all. While some defective distributions mentioned in this thesis could be used, the more interesting approach would be the use of so called cure rate models, which were not discussed in this thesis. Here the probability that an individual is "cured", so that failure becomes impossible, is explicitly modeled via a two-component mixture distribution.

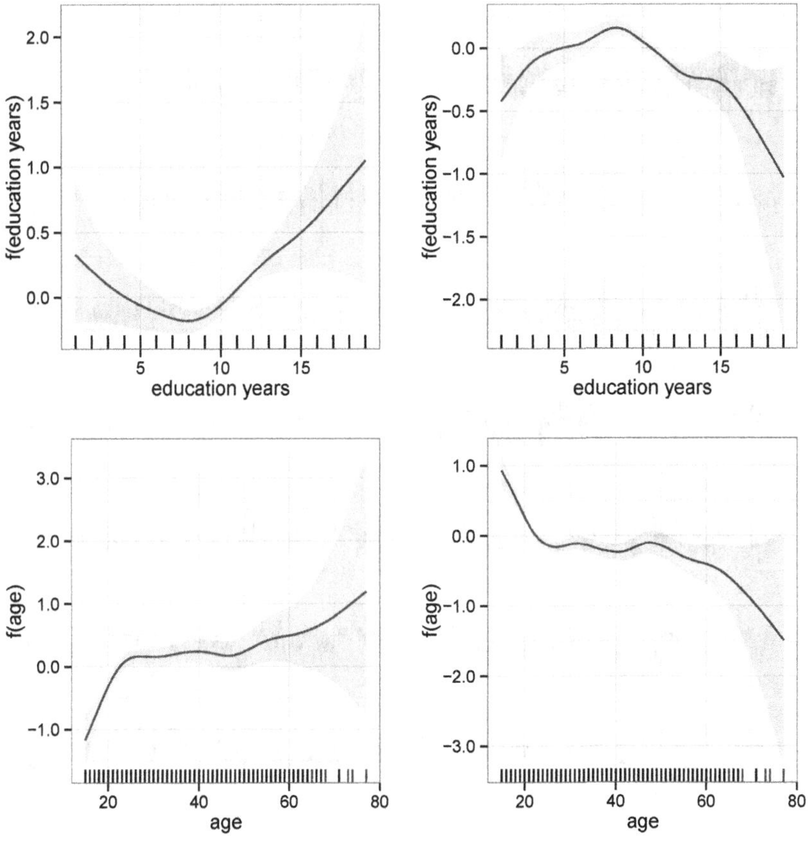

Figure 7.6: Estimated effects for both models with 5% and 95% posterior quantiles. The stripes represent unique observations. Left column: lognormal, right column: piecewise constant.

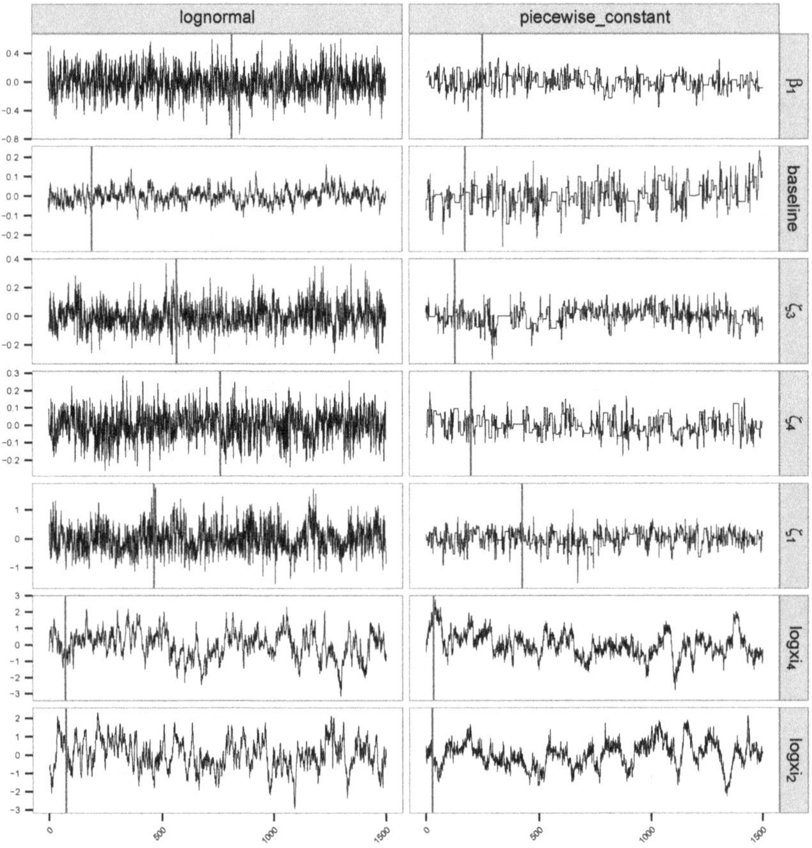

Figure 7.7: Selected sampling paths, both samplers for the last 1000 iterations. Blue vertical line is the effective number of draws. As can be seen, acceptance rates are low for piecewise constant model and mixing is better for the lognormal model. Note that all parameters have been centred for visualization purposes. Convergence for the smoothing variances is slow.

8 Summary and Outlook

Bayesian methods for the analysis of failure time data in continuous and discrete time using P-splines have been presented and applied. The sampling schemes can be summarized in the following way: (1) Sampling schemes where by introduction of latent variables Gaussian conditionals are obtained, then using the basic sampling scheme for the Gaussian likelihood. (2) Sampling schemes using IWLS proposals when full conditionals are not conditional conjugate. It turned out that with these samplers a broad range of models can be estimated with relative ease.

In the applications, the methods were applied. For the first application, IWLS proposals were tried out in connection with a data augmentation sampling scheme for the grouped Cox model. The performance of this sampler was found to be acceptable, the standard sampler using sampling scheme 3 showed some problems which could not be resolved. For the second application the piecewise constant model was estimated via completion Gibbs samplers. The mixing of the lognormal sampler was found to be satisfactory. The mixing of the piecewise constant sampler based on IWLS proposals was found to be improvable but good enough to base inferences on. In all cases smoothing variances converged slowly.

There are several possible directions for future research. Due to the often mentioned Poisson likelihood, a worthwile perspective might be to apply further methods for the Poisson likelihood. For example, a data augmentation scheme for the Poisson distribution has been developed by Frühwirth-Schnatter et al. (2009) using a normal mixture as approximation for two introduced latent variables. This approximation might be used directly or might be used as a proposal distribution for Metropolis-Hastings updates. Wang et al. (2012a) use a completion Gibbs sampler for interval-censored data where two latent Poisson variables are introduced, one of which is distributed as $Z_i \sim \mathscr{P}([H_0(r_i) - H_0(l_i)]\exp(\eta_i))$. An interesting approach would be to use P-splines for $H_0(t)$ instead of $h_0(t)$. The function would have to be restricted to be nonincreasing, this can in fact be achieved for P-splines by restricting the coefficients to be nonincreasing. This approach would have the advantage of not requiring numerical integration. The baseline could easily be obtained by standard formulae for the derivatives of P-splines. In a related note, other functions might be used for the log-baseline to bypass numerical intergration for acceptance steps. An interesting idea might be to use a weighted mixture of hazards; Komárek et al. (2005) use an approach similar to P-splines where a penalized mixture distribution is used for modeling of the log failure times. In their approach, the means of the component distribution are treated like knots and the mixture weights are penalized. This approach might be used for the log-baseline hazard, using e.g. a penalized mixture of Weibull hazards.

For failure time modeling, the data collection is often very important. An interesting research topic might be modeling techniques that correct for bias resulting from this by using the methods of this thesis, for example by using flexible measurement error models or a flexible multiple imputation algorithm to counteract heaping. The probit model might be an interesting choice, heteroskedasty might be introduced, for example variance might be related nonlinearly to the time difference between the interview and the beginning of exposure of failure.

Natural extensions are furthermore multiple modes of failure and recurrent failures. Extending the models to multiple modes of failure is straightforward in the discrete case; instead of models for binary data, models for polytomous data can be used. For continuous data, this is not straightforward and the modeling framework is somewhat different in this context. For recurrent failure models the situation is similar: Discrete time models for recurrent failures are often based around standard random effect models, while for continuous time again a different modeling framework is necessary, here counting process notation, as shortly discussed in the context of martingale residuals, is very useful.

Other approaches would be to research and compare alternative priors for variance parameters and different functions for the hazard rate in combination with P-splines. Alternatives to the relative risk hazard which have been suggested (Sun

2006, pp. 19–20) are the proportional odds model

$$\frac{G(t_i)}{1+G(t_i)} = \exp(-\eta_i)\frac{G_0(t_i)}{1+G_0(t_i)}$$

and the additive hazards model

$$h(t|\eta_i) = h_0(t_i) + \eta_i,$$

which could be analyzed by adjusting the methods of this thesis. For discrete time there have been suggestions of specialized response functions accounting for the nature of failure time data. Promising is the response function

$$P(T = t|T \geq t) = 1 - (1 + \zeta \exp(\eta))^{-1/\zeta}, \tag{8.1}$$

used by Hess (2009) for discrete failure time data. The function 8.1 fits heavily skewed data well and nests the response function of the grouped Cox as special case, inference could be carried out using IWLS proposals.

Appendix A: Description of R Function

To run the Gibbs sampler, a function was implemented in R. The necessary scripts are available on a CD appended to this thesis. The functions take are optimized exclusively for the applications and might not generalize well. The usage is outlined here. It should be noted that regarding computational speed, the functions could probably be improved. Several packages are necessary to run the functions:

- `Matrix` (Bates and Maechler 2013) for sparse matrix implementation which was essentiel for efficient computation and storing of B-spline design matrices.
- `splines` (R Core Team 2013) for fast creation of basis function matrices. The package conviently outputs sparse matrices
- `rtruncnorm` for draws from the truncated normal distribution as discussed in section 5
- `Rcpp` (Eddelbuettel and François 2011) this package provides a R interface to implement simple C++ functions which give computational advantages[1]
- `RcppArmadillo` (Eddelbuettel and Sanderson 2014) this package includes some functions necessary for fast matrix manipluation via rcpp
- `reshape2` this implements the melt function essential for fast creation of offsets for the piecewise constant sampler

Furthermore for the `rcpp` package installation of the program `Rtools` is necessary. The functions are implemented in the following files:

- `functions.R`
- `gibbs_all.R`
- `cppfunctions.cpp`

The file `functions.R` contains supporting functions implemented directly in R, the file `cppfunctions.cpp` contains supporting functions implemented in R via the rcpp package, the file `gibbs_all.R` contains the function `gibbs_all` used for estimation. The file

[1]Faster execution speeds could be possible using this more.

`main.R` can be adjusted for sourcing. After sourcing these files the function can be used if all pre-requisites are installed. The function takes the following arguments for all hazards, in brackets default values are given:

`Z`	design matrix
`Z.splines`	design matrix for splines
`r`(1000)	number of iterations
`beta0.Precision` (**0**)	prior precision of fixed effects
`beta0`	prior mean of fixed effects
`l.vector`	vector of degrees for splines
`d.vector`	vector of difference penalty for splines
`inter.act.list`	list for interactios
`lambda.start` (0.05)	start value for spline precision
`m.vector` (30)	vector for number of knots
`hyper.a0.vector` (0.0001)	vector of hyperparameter a0 for splines variances
`hyper.b0.vector (0.0001)`	vector of hyperparameter b0 for splines variances
`hazard`	hazard as string: available are piecewise_constant,lognormal, probit, cloglog, cloglog.poisson (for cloglog via Poisson data augmentation)
`just.objekts`(FALSE)	boolean indicating if gibbs sampler should only be run to give out objekts such as design matrices for splines

It is always assumes that there is a constant, if no design matrix for fixed effects is given, it is created. If a design matrix for fixed effects is given and contains no column of ones, a column one will be created. Counting for all basis function matrices start with first column of will.splines, followed by the basis matrices for varying coefficient terms. The list `inter.act.list` is organized as follows: Entries consist of matrices where the first column is effect modifier and the right column is the interaction variable. Following arguments are specific for discrete time models:

`Z`	design matrix
`y`	vector of failure indicators
`time.var`	variable giving process time
`time.blocked`	boolean indicating if seasonal and baseline hazard parameters are sampled in one block
`seas.var`	variable of time measurements, from 1 to maximal measurement of historical time
`per`	period length
`time.blocked`	boolean indicating seasonal coefficients and baseline hazard paramater are updated blockwise

Seasonal variables could also be used for continuous time, but this has not been tested. For the lognormal and piecewise constant model, interval censoring is assumed. Following arguments are specific for these hazard:

`upper`	vector of upper interval boundaries for failure time
`lower`	vector of upper interval boundaries for failure time
`res.var.a0` 0.001	hyperparameter a for the residual variance
`res.var.b0` 0.001	hyperparameter b for the residual variance

The first entries of d.vector and m.vector for the piecewise constant model are reserved for the baseline hazard. The function returns a list with the following objects:

`gamma`	list with matrices of B-spline coefficients with
`beta`	matrix of coefficients for fixed effects
`taus`	matrix of smoothing variances
`spline.design.mat`	list of entries necessary for plotting of splines

Furthermore, for the piecewise constant model, the function returns the list `baseline`, containing a matrix of regression coefficients, a vector of smoothing variances for the baseline coefficients and a vector of knots. For the lognormal model, the vector `sigma` containing the squared shape parameter σ^2 is given out. Splines can be plotted via the function plot.splines which can be found in `functions.R`.

In the following an example for a function call for discrete time is given:

```
gibbs.splines(Z=Z,id=data$id,per=12,seas.var=data$season,
time.var=data$t, hazard="probit", r=r,y=data$y,
Z.splines=Z.splines,inter.act.list=inter.act.list,
lambda.start=0.1, l.vector=c(3,3,3,3,3,3,3,3),
d.vector=c(2,2,2,2,2,2,2,2,2))
```

It has been observed that the start parameter `lambda.start` is influental regarding acceptance rates, if the function is run with low acceptance rates changing this parameter often helps. All IWLS proposals are based around sampling scheme 2. The parameters for basis function coefficients are sampled using the standard sum to zero (over the sample) restriction.

Bibliography

Aalen, O., Ø. Borgan, and S. Gjessing (2008). *Survival and event history analysis: A process point of view*. New York: Springer.

Aitkin, M. and D. Clayton (1980). "The fitting of exponential, Weibull and extreme value distributions to complex censored survival data using GLIM". In: *Applied Statistics* 29, pp. 156–163.

Albert, J. H. and S. Chib (1993). "Bayesian analysis of binary and polychotomous response data". In: *Journal of the American Statistical Association* 88, pp. 669–679.

Andrews, D. F. and C. L. Mallows (1974). "Scale Mixtures of Normal Distributions". In: *Journal of the Royal Statistical Society. Series B (Methodological)* 36, pp. 99–102.

Aslanidou, H., D. K. Dey, and D. Sinha (1998). "Bayesian Analysis of Multivariate Survival Data Using Monte Carlo Methods". In: *Canadian Journal of Statistics* 26, pp. 33–38.

Banerjee, S. and B. P. Carlin (2004). "Parametric Spatial Cure Rate Models for Interval-Censored Time-to-Relapse Data". In: *Biometrics* 60, pp. 268–275.

Bates, D. and M. Maechler (2013). *Matrix: Sparse and Dense Matrix Classes and Methods*. R package version 1.1-1.1.

Bebbington, M., C.-D. Lai, and R. Zitikis (2006). "Useful periods for lifetime distributions with bathtub shaped hazard rate functions." In: *IEEE Transactions on Reliability* 55, pp. 245–251.

Berg, G. J. Van den (2001). "Duration models: specification, identification and multiple durations". In: *Handbook of Econometrics*. Ed. by J. Heckman and E. Leamer. Vol. 5. Amsterdam: Elsevier, pp. 3380–3460.

Blossfeld, H.-P. and G. Rohwer (2002). *Techniques of event history modeling: New approaches to causal analysis*. 2nd ed. Mahwah: Lawrence Erlbaum.

Blossfeld, H.-P., H. G. Roßbach, and J. von Maurice (2011). "Education as a Lifelong Process: The German National Educational Panel Study (NEPS)". In: *Zeitschrift für Erziehungswissenschaft*, pp. 19–34.

Boor, C. de (2001). *A Practical Guide to Splines*. New York: Springer.

Brezger, A. and S. Lang (2006). "Generalized structured additive regression based on Bayesian P-splines". In: *Computational Statistics & Data Analysis* 50, pp. 967–991.

Cameron, A. C. and P. K. Trivedi (2005). *Microeconometrics: Methods and applications*. Cambridge: Cambridge University Press.

Carlin, B. and T. Louis (2011). *Bayesian Methods for Data Analysis, Third Edition*. Boca Raton: Taylor & Francis.

Cowles, M. K. and B. P. Carlin (1996). "Markov Chain Monte Carlo Convergence Diagnostics: A Comparative Review". In: *Journal of the American Statistical Association* 91, pp. 883–904.

Cox, D. R. (1972). "Regression Models and Life-Tables". In: *Journal of the Royal Statistical Society. Series B (Methodological)* 34, pp. 187–220.

Cox, D. R. and D. Oakes (1984). *Analysis of survival data*. London: Chapman and Hall.

Crowder, M. (2001). *Classical Competing Risks*. Boca Raton: Taylor & Francis.

Cumbus, C., P. Damien, and S. Walker (1996). *Sampling truncated poisson and multivariate normal densities via the gibbs sampler*. Technical Report. University of Michigan Business School.

Dellaportas, P. and G. O. Roberts (2003). "An introduction to MCMC". In: *Spatial Statistics and Computational Methods*. Ed. by J. Moller. New York: Springer, pp. 1–42.

Devroye, L. (1986). *Non-uniform random variate generation*. New York: Springer.

Diekmann, A. and P. Mitter (1983). "The "Sickle-Hypothesis": A Time-Dependent Poisson Model with Applications to Deviant Behaviour and Occupational Mobility". In: *Journal of Mathematical Sociology* 9, pp. 85–101.

Dierckx, P. (2006). *Curve and surface splitting with splines*. Oxford: Clarendon Press.

Dunson, D. B. and A. H. Herring (2004). "Bayesian latent variable models for mixed discrete outcomes". In: *Biostatistics* 6, pp. 11–25.

Eddelbuettel, D. and R. François (2011). "Rcpp: Seamless R and C++ Integration". In: *Journal of Statistical Software* 40, pp. 1–18.

Eddelbuettel, D. and C. Sanderson (2014). "RcppArmadillo: Accelerating R with high-performance C++ linear algebra". In: *Computational Statistics and Data Analysis* 71, pp. 1054–1063.

Eilers, P. H. C. and B. D. Marx (1996). "Flexible smoothing with B-splines and penalties". In: *Statistical Science* 11, pp. 89–121.

— (2010). "Splines, knots, and penalties". In: *Wiley Interdisciplinary Reviews: Computational Statistics* 2, pp. 637–653.

Fahrmeir, L. and T. Kneib (2011). *Bayesian smoothing and regression for longitudinal, spatial and event history data.* Oxford: Oxford University Press.

Fahrmeir, L. and G. Tutz (2001). *Multivariate statistical modelling based on generalized linear models.* 2nd ed. New York: Springer.

Fahrmeir, L., T. Kneib, S. Lang, and B. Marx (2013). *Regression: Models, Methods and Applications.* Heidelberg: Springer.

Fahrmeir, L. and S. Lang (2000). "Bayesian Inference for Generalized Additive Mixed Models Based on Markov Random Field Priors". In: *Journal of the Royal Statistical Society. Series C* 50, pp. 201–220.

Fleming, T. R. and D. P. Harrington (1991). *Counting processes and survival analysis.* New York: Wiley.

Flinn, C. and J. Heckman (1982). "Models for the Analysis of Labor Force Dynamics". In: *Advances in Econometrics* 1, pp. 35–95.

Frühwirth-Schnatter, S., R. Frühwirth, L. Held, and H. Rue (2009). "Improved auxiliary mixture sampling for hierarchical models of non-Gaussian data". In: *Statistics and Computing* 19, pp. 479–492.

Gamerman, D. and H. Lopes (2006). *Markov Chain Monte Carlo: Stochastic Simulation for Bayesian Inference.* 2nd ed. Boca Raton: Taylor & Francis.

Gamerman, D. (1997). "Sampling from the posterior distribution in generalized linear mixed models". In: *Statistics and Computing* 7, pp. 57–68.

Geisser, S. and W. F. Eddy (1979). "A Predictive Approach to Model Selection". In: *Journal of the American Statistical Association* 74, p. 153.

Gelfand, A. E. and D. K. Dey (1994). "Bayesian Model Choice: Asymptotics and Exact Calculations". In: *Journal of the Royal Statistical Society. Series B (Methodological)* 56, pp. 501–514.

Gelfand, A. (1996). "Model determination using sampling-based methods". In: *Markov Chain Monte Carlo in Practice*. Ed. by W. Gilks, S. Richardson, and D. Spiegelhalter. London: Chapman & Hall, pp. 145–162.

Gelfand, A. E. and S. K. Ghosh (1998). "Model Choice: A Minimum Posterior Predictive Loss Approach". In: *Biometrika* 85, pp. 1–11.

Gelman, A. (2006). "Prior distributions for variance parameters in hierarchical models". In: *Bayesian Analysis* 1, pp. 1–19.

Gelman, A., J. Hwang, and A. Vehtari (2013). "Understanding predictive information criteria for Bayesian models". In: *Statistics and Computing*, pp. 1–20.

Geweke, J. (1991). "Efficient simulation from the multivariate normal and student-t distributions subject to linear constraints and the evaluation of constraint probabilities". In: *Computing Science and Statistics: Proceedings of the 23rd Symposium on the Interface*. Fairfax Station: Interface Foundation, pp. 571–578.

Greene, W. H. (2012). *Econometric analysis*. 7th ed. Boston: Prentice Hall.

Gustafson, P. (1997). "Large Hierarchical Bayesian Analysis of Multivariate Survival Data". In: *Biometrics* 53, pp. 230–242.

Hanson, T. E. (2006). "Inference for Mixtures of Finite Polya Tree Models". In: *Journal of the American Statistical Association* 101, pp. 1548–1565.

Hastie, T. and R. Tibshirani (1993). "Varying-Coefficient Models". In: *Journal of the Royal Statistical Society. Series B (Methodological)* 55, pp. 757–796.

— (2000). "Bayesian Backfitting". In: *Statistical Science* 15, pp. 196–223.

Hastie, T., R. Tibshirani, and J. H. Friedman (2009). *The elements of statistical learning: Data mining, inference, and prediction*. 2nd ed. New York: Springer.

Heckman, J. J. and B. Singer (1984). "Econometric duration analysis". In: *Journal of Econometrics* 24, pp. 63–132.

Hennerfeind, A. (2006). "Bayesian nonparametric regression for survival and event history data". PhD thesis. Ludwig-Maximilians-Universität München.

Hennerfeind, A., A. Brezger, and L. Fahrmeir (2006). "Geoadditive Survival Models". In: *Journal of the American Statistical Association* 101, pp. 1065–1075.

Henschel, V., J. Engel, D. Hölzel, and U. Mansmann (2009). "A semiparametric Bayesian proportional hazards model for interval censored data with frailty effects". In: *BMC Medical Research Methodology* 9, p. 9.

Hess, W. (2009). *A Flexible Hazard Rate Model for Grouped Duration Data*. Technical Report. Lund University.

Holford, T. (1980). "The analysis of rates and of survivorship using log-linear models". In: *Biometrics* 36, pp. 299–305.

Ibrahim, J. G., M. H. Chen, and S. Debajyoti (2001a). "Criterion-based methods for Bayesian model assessment". In: *Statistica Sinica* 11, pp. 419–443.

Ibrahim, J. G., M.-H. Chen, and D. Sinha (2001b). *Bayesian survival analysis*. New York: Springer.

Kalbfleisch, J. D. and R. L. Prentice (2002). *The statistical analysis of failure time data*. 2nd ed. New York: Wiley.

Kalbfleisch, J. D. (1979). "Non-parametric Bayesian Analysis of Survival Time Data". In: *Journal of the Royal Statistical Society, Series B* 40, pp. 214–221.

Kalbfleisch, J. D. and R. L. Prentice (1973). "Marginal Likelihoods Based on Cox's Regression and Life Model". In: *Biometrika* 60, pp. 256–278.

Kass, R. E., B. P. Carlin, A. Gelman, and R. M. Neal (1998). "Markov Chain Monte Carlo in Practice: A Roundtable Discussion". In: *The American Statistician* 52, pp. 93–100.

Klein, J. P. and M. L. Moeschberger (2003). *Survival analysis: Techniques for censored and truncated data*. 2nd ed. New York: Springer.

Kneib, T. and A. Hennerfeind (2008). "Bayesian semi parametric multi-state models". In: *Statistical Modelling* 8, pp. 169–198.

Kneib, T. (2006). "Mixed model based inference in structured additive regression". PhD thesis. Ludwig-Maximilians-Universität München.

Knorr-Held, L. (1999). "Conditional Prior Proposals in Dynamic Models". In: *Scandinavian Journal of Statistics* 26, pp. 129–144.

Komárek, A., E. Lesaffre, and J. F. Hilton (2005). "Accelerated Failure Time Model for Arbitrarily Censored Data With Smoothed Error Distribution". In: *Journal of Computational and Graphical Statistics* 14, pp. 726–745.

Konrath, S. (2013). "Bayesian regularization in regression models for survival data". PhD thesis. Ludwig-Maximilians-Universität München.

Laird, N. and D. Olivier (1981). "Covariance Analysis of Censored Survival Data Using Log-linear Analysis Techniques". In: *Journal of the American Statistical Association* 76, pp. 231–240.

Lambert, P. and P. H. C. Eilers (2005). "Bayesian proportional hazards model with time-varying regression coefficients: A penalized Poisson regression approach." In: *Statistics in Medicine* 24, pp. 3977–3989.

Lang, S. and A. Brezger (2004). "Bayesian P-Splines". In: *Journal of Computational and Graphical Statistics* 13, pp. 183–212.

Lang, S., N. Umlauf, P. Wechselberger, K. Harttgen, and T. Kneib (2014). "Multilevel structured additive regression". In: *Statistics and Computing* 24, pp. 223–238.

Lawless, J. F. (2003). *Statistical models and methods for lifetime data.* 2nd ed. New York: Wiley.

Liu, C. (2004). "Robit Regression: A Simple Robust Alternative to Logistic and Probit Regression". In: *Applied Bayesian Modeling and Causal Inference from an Incomplete-Data Perspective.* Ed. by A. Gelman and X. L. Meng. New York: Wiley, pp. 227–238.

McCulloch, C. and S. Searle (2001). *Generalized, Linear, and Mixed Models.* New York: Wiley.

Murthy, D., M. Xie, and R. Jiang (2004). *Weibull Models.* New York: Wiley.

O'Sullivan, F. (1986). "A Statistical Perspective on Ill-Posed Inverse Problems". In: *Statistical Science* 1, pp. 502–518.

Plummer, M., N. Best, K. Cowles, and K. Vines (2006). "CODA: Convergence Diagnosis and Output Analysis for MCMC". In: *R News* 6, pp. 7–11.

Polson, N. G. and J. G. Scott (2011). "Shrink Globally, Act Locally: Sparse Bayesian Regularization and Prediction". In: *Bayesian Statistics 9.* Ed. by

J. Bernardo, J. Bayarri, J. Berger, A. Dawid, and D. Heckerman. Oxford: Oxford University Press, pp. 501–538.

R Core Team (2013). *R: A Language and Environment for Statistical Computing*. R Foundation for Statistical Computing. Vienna, Austria.

Robert, C. P. (2001). *The Bayesian Choice: From Decision-Theoretic Foundations to Computational Implementation*. New York: Springer.

Robert, C. P. (1995). "Simulation of truncated normal variables". In: *Statistics and Computing* 5, pp. 121–125.

Robert, C. P. and G. Casella (2004). *Monte Carlo statistical methods*. 2nd ed. New York: Springer.

Roberts, G. (1996). "Markov chain concepts related to sampling algorithms". In: *Markov Chain Monte Carlo in Practice*. Ed. by W. Gilks, S. Richardson, and D. Spiegelhalter. London: Chapman & Hall, pp. 45–54.

Rosenthal, J. S. (2011). "Optimal Proposal Distributions and Adaptive MCMC". In: *Handbook of Markov Chain Monte Carlo*. Ed. by S. Brooks, A. Gelman, G. L. Jones, and X.-L. Meng. First. Chapman & Hall, CRC.

Rue, H. and L. Held (2005). *Gaussian Markov Random Fields: Theory and Applications*. Boca Raton: Taylor & Francis.

Schmidt, P. and A. D. Witte (1988). *Predicting Recidivism Using Survival Models*. New York: Springer.

Sha, N., M. G. Tadesse, and M. Vannucci (2006). "Bayesian variable selection for the analysis of microarray data with censored outcomes". In: *Bioinformatics* 22, pp. 2262–2268.

Spiegelhalter, S. D., N. G. Best, B. P. Carlin, and A. V. D. Linde (2002). "Bayesian measures of model complexity and fit". In: *Journal of the Royal Statistical Society: Series B (Statistical Methodology)* 64, pp. 583–639.

Sun, J. (2006). *The statistical analysis of interval-censored failure time data*. New York: Springer.

Tanner, M. A. and W. H. Wong (1987). "The Calculation of Posterior Distributions by Data Augmentation". In: *Journal of the American Statistical Association* 82, pp. 528–540.

Thall, P. F., L. H. Wooten, and N. M. Tannir (2005). "Monitoring event times in early phase clinical trials: some practical issues." In: *Clinical Trials* 2, pp. 467–478.

Therneau, T. and P. Grambsch (2000). *Modeling Survival Data: Extending the Cox Model*. New York: Springer.

Tierney, L. (1996). "Introduction to general state-space Markov chain theory". In: *Markov Chain Monte Carlo in Practice*. Ed. by W. Gilks, S. Richardson, and D. Spiegelhalter. London: Chapman & Hall, pp. 59–74.

Trautmann, H., D. Steuer, O. Mersmann, and B. Bornkamp (2012). *truncnorm: Truncated normal distribution*. R package version 1.0-6.

Vehtari, A. and J. Ojanen (2012). "A survey of Bayesian predictive methods for model assessment, selection and comparison". In: *Statistics Surveys* 6, pp. 142–228.

Venables, W. N. and B. D. Ripley (2002). *Modern Applied Statistics with S*. 4th ed. New York: Springer.

Wang, L., X. I. Lin, and B. Cai (2012a). "Bayesian Semiparametic Regression Analysis of Interval-Censored data with Monotone Splines". In: *Interval-Censored Time-to-Event Data: Methods and Applications*. Ed. by D. Chen, J. Sun, and K. Peace. Boca Raton: Taylor & Francis, pp. 149–165.

Wang, X., A. Sinha, J. Yan, and M.-H. Chen (2012b). "Bayesian Inference of Interval-Censored data". In: *Interval-Censored Time-to-Event Data: Methods and Applications*. Ed. by D. Chen, J. Sun, and K. Peace. Boca Raton: Taylor & Francis, pp. 167–195.

Wienke, A. (2010). *Frailty Models in Survival Analysis*. Boca Raton: Taylor & Francis.

Yavuz, A. C. and P. Lambert (2011). "Smooth estimation of survival functions and hazard ratios from interval-censored data using Bayesian penalized B-splines." In: *Statistics in medicine* 30, pp. 75–90.